Empath and Psychic Abilities

A Complete Guide to Awakening Your Powers and Protecting Your Energy

Camilla Driscoll

© **Copyright 2022–All rights reserved.**

The content contained within this book may not be reproduced, duplicated or transmitted without direct written permission from the author or the publisher.

Under no circumstances will any blame or legal responsibility be held against the publisher, or author, for any damages, reparation, or monetary loss due to the information contained within this book, either directly or indirectly.

Legal Notice:

This book is copyright protected. It is only for personal use. You cannot amend, distribute, sell, use, quote or paraphrase any part, or the content within this book, without the consent of the author or publisher.

Disclaimer Notice:

Please note the information contained within this document is for educational and entertainment purposes only. All effort has been executed to present accurate, up to date, reliable, complete information. No warranties of any kind are declared or implied. Readers acknowledge that the author is not engaged in the rendering of legal, financial, medical or professional advice. The content within this book has been derived from various sources. Please consult a licensed professional before attempting any techniques outlined in this book.

By reading this document, the reader agrees that under no circumstances is the author responsible for any losses, direct or indirect, that are incurred as a result of the use of the information contained within this document, including, but not limited to, errors, omissions, or inaccuracies.

Table of Contents

Introduction 1

Chapter 1: What Is a Psychic Empath? 5

Chapter 2: Are You a Psychic Empath? 13

Chapter 3: What Kind of Empath Are You? 20

Chapter 4: Myths and Mysteries 28

Chapter 5: The Science Behind Being an Empath 36

Chapter 6: All the Clairs Explained 41

Chapter 7: Psychic Protection 48

Chapter 8: Psychic Self-Care 70

Chapter 9: Strengthening Psychic Skills 85

Chapter 10: Psychic Awakenings 91

Chapter 11: Working With the Universe 95

Chapter 12: Out in the World 100

Chapter 13: Using Your Gifts 105

Chapter 14: Parenting an Empath Child 109

Chapter 15: Tips and Tricks For When Everything Feels Hard 114

Conclusion 118

References 123

Introduction

Huge, adorable, chocolate-brown eyes peered up at me, with sweet hairy eyebrows raised in distress. Candy, a beautiful and gentle golden Labrador, had been behaving very strangely. At times, she would snap and growl at her very loving owner, but nobody knew why. Most of the time, she was perfectly lovely and well behaved. Her sudden aggressive behavior made no sense. In desperation, the family called me. They admitted they were considering having Candy put down because they were concerned the dog could be a danger around their small children.

When I met Candy and her family, the issue was immediately clear to me— Candy was acting out because of a sweater. Candy's owner recently started wearing a bright new orange sweater and I could see that the sweater was setting off the usually sweet dog. Candy had been hurt as a puppy by her breeder, who wore a sweater just like this one. When Candy saw June's new sweater, she was sent back to a time when she felt very lonely and afraid. This triggered Candy's sudden aggressive behavior. The typically sweet dog's growling was only confusing if you didn't understand or know the context. So I told June not to wear the sweater anymore around Candy and I explained what I saw.

"You will not believe it," June gushed on the phone to me a few weeks later. "Candy has been fine ever since I got rid of that sweater!"

This did not surprise me. But of course, how was June to know that the sweater was to blame for her poor dog's sudden aggression? From the outside, Candy simply seemed a bit "off" and unpredictable, dangerous even. But the poor dog was just extremely triggered and very frightened. I was so happy I was able to understand the cause of Candy's strange behavior and figure out the trigger. It gives me extreme solace that I was able to save that sweet pup's life as well as help that family out.

I have been dialed in to my abilities for quite some time now. I believe I inherited this gift from my mom, who is what is known as a psychic empath. My mom only started understanding her skills late in life, after a lot of pain and suffering, attracting all the wrong sorts of people. Thank goodness I learned from her, and learned early.

A lot of people look down on empaths. They paint us as overly emotional, too sensitive, and a range of other cruel and belittling terms. It's easy to label and dismiss something you don't understand and have never experienced. And yet there are so many of us out there who desperately need to understand who we are, what is going on, and how to handle it all. Sadly, many psychic empaths only come to these realizations after a lot of pain and suffering, but it does not need to be this way.

Accepting my gifts was a huge learning curve. It's a journey I need to share with you because if you are reading this, you know something is going on- you are likely experiencing life quite a lot more intensely than others- and maybe you could do with some help and support.

We need to shake free of the unhelpful and limiting stigma attached to being who we are. There is no shame in having an ability like this. Quite the opposite. And yes, the heightened anxiety, roller-coaster emotions, and overwhelming influx of information we get from the world and people around us can be super confusing. At first we often think these thoughts and feelings belong to us, but they don't. The minute you learn to shut that flow off at will and to pull your energy protectively around you rather than letting it spiderweb out into everyone else's auras, the peace is clear. When you experience the sense of calm that comes from honing and developing your gift, you'll realize that a lot of the intense energy you've been carrying around for so long is not yours.

Even better, once you learn how to work with your ability, you can pick and choose when you use it and with whom. I prefer to keep the energies of other people and places out of my experience most of the time. People around me can carry such an overwhelming amount of data, and I rarely want that muddying up my day or my heart and head. Animals are different, though. I love dipping into their clear, pure energy. It's generally so simple and unadulterated. There is no agenda. There is no "monkey mind" ego chatter or lack of worth. Things are just however they are.

Most of the time, I use my psychic empath gifts to understand animals. As a fauna empath and clairsentient, I "see" energy rather than hear or feel it to help these beautiful beings who otherwise don't have much of a voice. (Actually, animals do have a very clear voice but, understandably, most humans don't know what exactly they're trying to say). While people and animals live fairly harmoniously side by side, the relationship often works due to the grace and loyalty of the animal. It amazes me how these beings fit their lives around humans, an entirely different species, and give us so much unquestioning love and support. I love being around my two very nurturing and affectionate dogs.

My son and my amazingly supportive husband are the other important elements in my life. I can already see my son showing signs that he is going to need empath training. Thank goodness I can be there for him so that he can learn how to live in this world and be minimally harmed by his gifts. My gratitude for understanding the gift of being an empath is boundless, and as my son develops, we are finding a lot of commonality and shared experiences that bind the connection between us closer. It's good to be around others who "get" you.

I have learned so much that helps me in my everyday life. My regular ocean swims and beach walks use water energy to ground and purify me. Meditation practices have given me the ability to calm and focus my mind no matter where I am and what I am doing. I have used these techniques and many others to strengthen my control over myself and my abilities. My deep connection to nature and my daily immersion in it on my long nature hikes soothe my soul and give me much needed space from a very busy world. All these little things are what I so desperately need as a psychic empath to stay safe, stable, and grounded. What might you need to ground yourself and grow your gifts?

There is so much you can do to strengthen, master, and manage the gifts that you have. You are a person capable of great strength and great love. You are innately worthy and full of inner wisdom and potential.

I hope what I have to share, all the wisdom—and the practical little tips and exercises—are going to help you along your way to self-mastery. Empaths have so much to offer the world, and psychic empaths are a true treasure.

Let's show you how to access these gifts safely and why you really want to do so.

Chapter 1:
What Is a Psychic Empath?

Empaths did not come into this world to be victims, we came to be warriors. Be brave. Stay strong. We need all hands on deck. —Anthon St. Maarten

Imagine a line.

On one end is the absence of any sensory input—no sight, sound, taste, touch, sight, nothing. You are an island in space, not even connected to any other by land or water. Because there is no input of any sort, there is also very little progress or learning.

Now see that same line stretch into the distance with a beautiful rainbow gradation of color—each hue representing a slightly different version of itself. At the other end, is, well, who knows, maybe God? Because this end of the spectrum is all-encompassing, all-knowing, omniscient.

Most people fall somewhere in between on this line. A basic level of empathy is required to be a social being. We all have many thoughts and feelings within us that drive our choices and actions. For us to act cohesively and cooperatively, we need to have some idea of what other people are thinking and feeling. The better we can do this, the better our chances of survival will be. So it can be said that highly developed empathy is an indication of a highly evolved social being. In order for the individual to survive, the whole group needs to survive, and perhaps this is the main reason we develop empathy.

Empathy is a social skill that we all have in differing degrees. It's the ability to understand what another being is experiencing on many levels. Furthermore, it is the ability to understand what someone's experience means and how they may be feeling as a result. Empathy is way more than just sympathizing, which has more to do with thinking about another person's experience based on your own experience. Empathy is fully immersing yourself in the other person (or beings, because you can empathize with animals, plants, or any life form you choose) and their experience.

Empathy is the sincere attempt to

- Feel into what the other feels, or at least understand this feeling.
- Understand what the other thinks.

In that sense, it is a higher form of communication. It goes beyond mere words although words can be used to describe thoughts and feelings and to gain common understanding.

Researchers have noted tiny newborns displaying empathy, crying in response to another baby's cry (Field et al., 2007). So we can say that empathy is wired into us so that we may all get along better together.

Perhaps sociopaths and extreme narcissists fall towards the not particularly empathetic end of the spectrum, which makes them socially dangerous. But the rest of us will be somewhere farther along the learning curve. We will be able to experience some level of empathy for others and display caring, nurturing, supportive, and compassionate behavior toward them as a result.

On the far end of the spectrum, we have highly developed empaths who absorb too much input, and even farther along the spectrum there are the psychic empaths who absorb information about others in ways that the rational mind cannot explain.

Let's delve a little deeper into the differences.

Emotionally Blinded

In the last century or so, we have emotionally disabled ourselves without realizing it. Our emotions are a very necessary part of our human experience. Just as we have physical senses that tell us about the outside world, we have emotional senses that tell us about our inner worlds. When something is off, unbalanced, or needing attention in our physical world, we feel physical discomfort or even pain, and the same happens with our emotional state.

But the problem is that the mind has become idolized above all else. Rationality, logic, and science have prevailed. This would be a good thing if it didn't mean that intuition and emotions were completely dismissed as unnecessary. It's a bit like saying now I have eyes so I don't need ears. We need all of our senses and abilities. Logic can supplement, but not replace emotion; one does not cancel the other out.

Toxic positivity has become the new black. Just smile and everything will be okay! Fake it till you make it! You know the drill. Do not show discomfort or too much emotion. Be in control at all times. Do not even admit to having any negative emotions. Emotions are weak! This whole "just suck it up" cult following has resulted in generations of people who do not know what they are feeling or why they feel the way they do. So many people avoid, deny, or suppress their feelings. These people do not know what to do with their feelings, so the bubbling emotions are bottled up until they finally leak out in toxic, inappropriate ways.

There are a lot of people going about their lives in emotional pain that they attempt to numb with work, drugs, alcohol, or other distractions. Sometimes these numbed out people will lash out at those closest to them, causing more pain all around them. All of this adds up to the walking emotionally wounded all around us. Anyone remotely sensitive to any of this will pick up on emotional chaos in every corner of their lives. This can turn into an emotional nightmare for empaths, especially if they don't know how to shut that kind of energy out.

Emotions and thoughts have an energy - they are extremely powerful. We can harness both energy and thoughts as tools to learn how to use in order to avoid hurting ourselves. If you think about a tool such as a knife, you know it can be very useful when used correctly and very harmful when used carelessly; the same idea applies to our minds and hearts.

When we are shut down- numbing, avoiding, letting fear control us, and denying a vital part of ourselves- we are in danger of moving closer to the narcissistic, unaware side of the empathy spectrum.

When a person lacks empathy we may notice some or all of the following:

- Confusion or a lack of understanding of other people's emotions
- Avoidance of and struggle to cope with emotional situations
- Lack of understanding, sympathy, or patience
- An inability to listen to or understand another's perspective or opinion

- Lack of forgiveness
- Lack of compassion
- Lots of blaming
- High levels of criticism
- Frustration or anger with others
- An inability to understand how their behavior affects others

People like this often seem as if their emotional development and ability to communicate stopped in early childhood. Sometimes the traits above can manifest so strongly that they can constitute an "emotional disorder" diagnosis of narcissism and sociopathy. So it becomes clear why empathy and emotional mastery are so necessary.

We don't know exactly why some people are more empathic than others. Early childhood and learning experiences, genetics, brain wiring, and socialization are all a part of the picture. But it certainly does not help that as a society we have conditioned ourselves to become emotionally shut down and cut off. Part of making the world a safer place emotionally, for ourselves and for others, is the process of learning emotional mastery rather than avoidance.

We badly need to reframe how we think about emotions. When we start engaging with our emotions, becoming self-aware, and learning to identify and process our feelings, we don't simply help ourselves. We help everyone around us who are otherwise caught in the backlash of our unmanaged emotional storms.

Highly Sensitive People

A sensitive person will pick up on slightly more than average external data coming from others and Highly Sensitive People, or "HSPs," will feel even more into what is going on. For example, an HSP may feel a physical twinge in empathy when they see someone else's wound. An HSP might feel inexplicably down when confronted with a particular crowd of people.

Sensitive people are more responsive to all sorts of sensory input, including other people's emotions, and may struggle to not take others' feelings on board and then react badly themselves. A sensitive person's reaction to these external feelings depends on how well they've developed their own coping mechanisms. Sensitive people may get hurt easily and cry easily, but they may also laugh easily.

Increasingly, it has become recognized that a large number of people are simply more sensitive than others, to the degree that problems can develop for them with no coping or self-protection mechanism in place. Psychologists believe highly sensitive people (HSPs) have a more developed central nervous system, which is more sensitive to emotional, social, and physical stimuli. About 20% of the population are believed to function this way (Scott, 2022).

More developed nervous systems have upsides and downsides. If you are highly sensitive, your level of sensitivity can mean that you're extremely responsive to good things as well as bad. An HSP will feel joy deeply and peace intensely, and they will be easily and deeply moved by beauty in all its forms. HSPs can sometimes feel deep gratitude for the loveliness of the sky, or the tastiness of a good cookie. You may feel intense and overwhelming happiness when your friend gets the new job they've been gunning for, or when your sister buys her dream home. So while you feel everything more intensely, there are naturally bright sides to your sensitive nature.

However, with the good comes the bad. A chaotic place or an angry person will unsettle you way more than it would a less sensitive person. You can get overwhelmed by too much sensory input, such as a noisy crowd, a nightclub, being under bright lights, or touching Grandma's scratchy Christmas sweater. Violence and horror on the screen is often too intense for you, as is too much news or any media for that matter, so they have to be limited or avoided.

Sensitive people will often find themselves retreating from the world into a quiet, calm space, a darkened room, or out into the soothing surrounds of nature. It is not a bad thing to retreat from the world from time to time, although it may leave the less sensitive portion of the population a little confused as to why you've gone away. That's okay though- taking time to recharge can be your superpower if you learn how to manage it well.

Being an Empath

There is a difference between having basic empathy for another and being an empath. The first trait is expected of you as a person living in society. When someone lacks empathy or treats others without empathy, we sometimes call that narcissistic or sociopathic.

However, being an empath means that we have taken empathy to a whole new level. Being an empath means that we pick up on emotional, physical, and social cues in ways that cannot always be easily explained. Perhaps our brains are wired differently? Perhaps our senses are more keenly developed? All empaths are highly attuned to the emotional states of those around them. Some empaths are so developed that they can tune in to people far away or read the energetic signatures that strong emotions have left in places or on items.

A psychic, or intuitive, empath is someone who appears to pick up on information about others without any (or few) verbal or visual clues. Psychic empaths somehow appear to intuitively know what is going on at a level that is not obvious to others. Somebody with this ability will be able to reproduce this skill fairly consistently over time, which tells us that it is not a coincidence. Additionally, being a psychic empath has been the subject of ongoing research as scientists try to quantify it and pin it down.

There are many kinds of empaths, but what is clear is that, whether we're psychic empaths or not, if we know how to use our ability and protect our own hearts, minds, and souls in the process, then we can help ourselves and many others too. We have been gifted with superpowers of sharing and knowing, and anything that helps us understand ourselves, situations, and others better can be a very good thing if used wisely.

Chapter 2:
Are You a Psychic Empath?

I'm terrified about psychic people who have their little shops. I always walk across the street and go somewhere else. Imagine if one of them came out with their face all pale and said, "Hurry up and enjoy yourself." No one wants to know that. –Mads Mikkelsen

The psychic empath is a special breed. In a way the word "psychic" is a bit redundant because to be psychic, you first need to dial into empathy to a large degree. The ability to reach out with your energy—beyond the confines of yourself and your own mind, heart, and body- and to pick up information from the people, things, and places around you, means that you can't help but have a deeper level of compassion and understanding for others and for life.

When you are a psychic empath, you literally know what it feels like to be others because for a fleeting moment, you have stepped inside their lives and into their world. If psychic empathy is not one of the highest forms of empathy, I don't know what is.

The psychic part of this deal means that you are very skilled in picking up on information that most people are unaware of. You have an extrasensory ability that lets you know things that most people simply cannot explain.

I believe that all empaths have this psychic ability and that it can be developed just like a keen sense of smell is developed by Parisienne parfumiers or a sense of space and movement is refined by a gymnast. It does seem, however, that some people are extra gifted in naturally knowing how to use their skills. Perhaps this talent is genetic, and they are born with something extra- an additional set of sensory organs and skills? Scientists have not yet proven where psychic empath skills might come from. Certain specific types of environments bring out a psychic sense in people. Often traumatic or unsafe childhood (or life) experiences seem to force certain people to turn on a whole extra level of danger detectors, and this bleeds into the psychic space quite often.

The typical profile of a psychic empath will include some, if not all, of these things in various combinations:

- You have been through a deeply unsettling phase of life where you did not feel safe or settled.

- You are hyper aware of what other people are doing, saying, and also thinking and feeling.

- Your nerves often feel raw.

- Your mood has been (or is) all over the place with no clear trigger to explain why.

- Being alone is like balm to your soul. You are introverted and prefer your own company simply because it is less "noisy" on a psychic and empathic level.

- You may feel drawn to help others, and sometimes this is simply to reduce the pain you are picking up on and feeling from others.

- You can often feel nauseous or ill for no specific reason.

- Social situations can feel like a waking nightmare. A big crowd, a busy mall, or even a small party can feel just too much for you.

- You know things about people, places, and situations, and you can't always explain how you know. Often, you discover later on you are right about these impressions.

Most psychic empaths have gone through quite a few harrowing nightmare situations already. Our practical, factual world full of, quite frankly, damaged, unaware people is extremely triggering.

You may have been in several traumatic relationships by now. That's often a given, because while others may not understand us, they are attracted to our healing energies. People sense that with us they will find compassion, love, kindness, and understanding that they will not get anywhere else. For souls in deep pain, we are very attractive indeed. Even if in the process these suffering souls wreck and destroy the very people they need, they keep coming back for more.

It's possible that you have been diagnosed with a personality disorder. From the outside, the experience of a psychic empath can fit into the boxes of several personality disorders such as Bipolar Disorder or Borderline Personality Disorder. Perhaps you have been on anti-anxiety and anti-depressant medications for some time. These medications, by the way, can actually be an unexpected boon because many psych-related meds also shut down or dampen psychic ability. Honestly, you may need that break while you regroup and heal.

What will be a fact, regardless of any of the rest, is that for a large part of your life, you have been carrying some very heavy feelings. These are not the nice, happy ones- they will instead be a range of the worst kind. And you may think this is how everyone feels in life, but it truly is not. Life is not so hard for the less sensitive. Maybe that's why less sensitive people choose to stay that way.

You will have been told, or convinced, that there is something wrong with you on some level. You may think that what you are feeling is who you are or that it belongs to you, but often it does not. Unprotected, untrained psychic empaths naturally absorb the emotions around them like a sponge and have no filter or protection in this process. Depending on the person, they may not only absorb the emotions of those in the room, or area, but they may also pick up on energies and data in a space from long ago, or from far away. Psychic empaths may be able to tell what a person who wore that specific bracelet was feeling three centuries ago or what was on the mind of the fellow traveler who sat on the same bus seat a week ago. Sitting on a chair that a very depressed person just vacated, or drinking from a glass that an anxious person touched (even if it was washed) can impact you with whatever they were thinking and feeling.

Practical Exercise: Empath Rating

If you are still unsure where you fit in, and whether you are truly a psychic empath or not, try this analytical tool to help you out:

Criteria	Not really/sometimes/a lot
I feel a mixed bag of emotions when I am in a crowd of people.	
In conversations, I can clearly identify the subtle undercurrents of thought and	

emotion present in the other person.	
People often tell me I am a great listener.	
Strangers and friends feel comfortable sharing personal details with me.	
People like to be near me or touch me. They often say it makes them feel better.	
I have a calming effect on others.	
I often know what will happen before it does.	
I often know things about people, places, or situations that amaze others as I had no way of knowing that information.	
I would prefer to be alone, except for a very few special people who don't disturb me if they are around.	
A depressed, angry, ill, or fearful person can be overwhelming for me.	
I can "feel" or sense the energy from people, animals, and/or even inanimate objects	

like food and antiques.	
I often feel fatigued and have unexplainable aches and pains in my body.	
I often focus on the needs of others, even over my own.	
Violence, tragedy, or cruelty in TV shows, movies, newspapers and books is almost unbearable for me to read or watch.	
I often experience a variety of strong emotions in a single day. I can go from happiness, to anger, to sadness, to joy and more.	

If you answered "a lot" to more than seven of these, you are a psychic empath. Collect your badge and a suit of armor at the door because it is time to arm up and get ready. If you said "sometimes" to seven or more of these, you are an empath who can very likely develop some psychic skills.

The life of a psychic empath, without the knowledge and skills you need to navigate these extra abilities of yours, can look chaotic and hard. I know I have painted quite a bleak picture here, but I believe there we really need to face this head on. The time to tiptoe around the issue, doubt ourselves, denigrate our abilities, and explain all of our deep feelings away needs to be over yesterday. There is only one way through this situation that will work to transform you into the super powerful person you can be; you need to deal with the facts as they are. Only in that way can we discover the best way forward. Otherwise we are navigating in the mist.

I firmly believe that in time to come, when science and popular opinion eventually catches up with an understanding of psychic empaths, people may refer back to these times as the psychic dark ages. How dreadful to leave a person raw, unprotected, derided, and in pain, when this person is potentially one of the world's most useful healers and lightworkers. We are a needed resource in a damaged world.

This is why I am writing this book. The world needs us so desperately, and as things stand, too many psychic empaths are being hurt by and within the system we are here to help and heal. We never get the chance to shine our light, and we certainly don't get the vital support we need. It's a bit like killing off all the caterpillars and then complaining that there are no more butterflies.

Okay, so now I will show you how to hone and develop your gift in a tough world as a psychic empath. Let's start with the basics. What kind of empath are you?

Chapter 3:
What Kind of Empath Are You?

A human being has so many skins inside, covering the depths of the heart. We know so many things, but we don't know ourselves! Why, thirty or forty skins or hides, as thick and hard as an ox's or bear's, cover the soul. Go into your own ground and learn to know yourself there. —Meister Eckhart

To know who you are, as an empath, is the beginning of a beautiful journey of self-discovery and development.

Just like in life where we are all talented in a multitude of ways with all sorts of combinations of level and type of ability, this spread of skills also applies to psychic empaths. There are all-rounders, who can work within all categories, and there are those who have a specific facility for certain areas more than others. See if you can recognize yourself from this list:

- **Plant empaths** (or flora empaths) have the proverbial green thumb. What is more, you always seem to know what plant wants to be where in your home and where it will flourish and be happy. Being in nature and around flora is soothing and also inspires you to dig, root around, feed, water, and sometimes just sit in silent communion with plants, shrubs, trees, and even the weeds. You don't pick from a plant without a quiet request and giving thanks. You don't like to see damaged or dried up plants. Being in a forest, or green spot, helps you feel connected in a way you can't easily explain. The energy of plants can be can be calming to you, but also insistent.

- **Animal empaths** (or fauna empaths) can connect into an animal's unspoken needs, feelings, and thoughts. You are the horse, cat, bird, bunny, and dog "whisperers." Most people can read up on an animal's body language and infer certain things from an animal's messages. It is especially easy to do this with very social animals like dogs, for example, who are also quite "humanized" in many ways. An animal empath can read deeper into an animal's feelings than a typical person. Animal empaths might pick up on information that does not always make sense in human terms but makes complete sense to the animal they are tuning in to.

- **Geomantic empaths** find it quite easy to tune in to earth energy. They make great dowsers for water and other resources. They can feel the places on the planet where energy gathers or runs in channels, much like an acupuncturist knows where a person's energy meridians run on their bodies. A geomantic can also feel when the energy is wrong, off, blocked, or damaged in some way. Geomantic empaths may be the people active in the environmental conservation space. You will find geomantics living near rivers, waterfalls, oceans, and in lush parts of the world, if they have a choice. Cities and highly populated areas are particularly draining for geomantic empaths long term.

- **Precognitive empaths** are not too restricted by the bounds of time; they can easily connect into the time flow and tune into events from the past and future. Precogs will get a sense of what might happen, which often starts off as smaller flashes of the immediate future but with practice can see even further. That being said, future precognition can be very confusing even to the best developed empath. Each choice made will turn up a new pathway, and sometimes a precog gets to see many possibilities that will distill down as each action is taken or decision made. The future is very pliable and potentially changeable.

- **Telepathic empaths** find it fairly easy to pick up on thoughts, and are also quite good at conveying meaning using very few words or gestures. Telepaths might experience their gift as a sudden insight or aha moment, or by noticing a random thought that feels alien to them. Often these feelings come to telepaths because they have picked up on the mental noise around them and are open enough to literally download another person's mental mutterings.

- **Dream empaths** walk in our sleeping world and find it easy to control what happens there for themselves and sometimes for others. Dream empaths can lucid dream and have, with experience, learned to take their dreams seriously as harbingers or indicators of what needs to be known. These empaths can appear in your dreams and don't need to be lying next to you to do so. They can heal through dreams and comfort. They can help others make sense of and work through disturbing dreams.

- **Emotive empaths** tune in to emotions more readily than to thoughts. This is just another way of saying "empath," as most empaths are, in fact, emotive empaths.

- **Intuitive or claircognizant empaths** are likely the most common type of psychic empath- in fact these are really just other ways of saying "psychic empath." All empaths generally have a foundation of intuition and are able to tune into the feelings of others. So most empaths are first claircognizants and then also may have further gifts in the other categories. Claircognizants can tune into thoughts, feelings, needs, and problems without you having to say that much. Clairs and Intuitives make excellent therapists and healers of all kinds.

As you can see, there are many ways your psychic empath abilities can present and develop, and all can be very useful if you learn how to direct and manage them well.

Know Your Strengths

How can you know what kind of empath you are? The odds are that if one of the above categories speaks to you, that is where you fall. Often psychic empaths have abilities that overlap into other categories. Your empath label may not be clear cut, but it does not have to be. Just try to feel into what type of empath feels right for you. One or a few of these categories will resonate and look and sound very familiar. You will have an "aha, that's me" moment. It is as simple as that.

The reason you want to pick a type is mainly for your own development purposes because knowing your type will help you to focus your energies towards that specific strength. Contrary to what everyone says about how to grow your skills, it is always best to work on your strengths first. Working on what you are already good at will help you gain confidence and strength, because it does not take much to fine-tune these natural skills. Once you have upgraded a strength into a level of mastery that you are content with, you can then look at next steps.

It's a bit pointless, not to mention a bit disheartening and demotivating, to try to push your abilities into an area that is totally unfamiliar or not a strong point. The problem with doing this first is that it may take a long while to see any progress in an unknown area, and on the way, you may give up. This may mean you never get to finesse the strengths you already have. Strengthening your area of natural ability does not mean you completely ignore any parts of yourself or your life you want to develop in the long run. If you're naturally an emotive empath, but want to strengthen your less developed telepathic abilities, you can definitely learn to do that down the line.

Speak to Your Strengths

Consider what you could do to start developing your skill set even more. This will mainly involve spending time working in those areas that are your strengths. See below for ways to begin to really grow and develop your gifts:

Plant Empaths

Spend as much time as you can in and around the plant spirits you feel most at home with. Get to know your favorites by really focusing on a specific plant at a time. This means that you spend time with that plant. You meditate on that plant and you explore all of its benefits and uses. If safe to do so, you can drink the dried form of that plant in a tea and use its oils as perfume. Spend a week or more per plant type. If possible, get to know a specific plant within the type. Commune with it. Keep records of what you learn so that later on you don't forget or lose track. Each plant has its own energy or spirit, and has a lot to teach you beyond the simple uses and benefits.

Spending time in your garden with hands and feet in the soil, or with your potted plants if you have no garden space, is not only soothing for you but will deepen your relationship with the plant world.

If you can, find a botanist, herbalist, or mushroom expert to go foraging with so that you can learn from them. Always spend time energetically linking with any plant to ask permission before you pick or harvest any part of it. If you are tuned into plant energy, you will always gZet a clear yes or no when you ask. If it is a no, move on to another plant.

Be aware that all plant life communes with each other in ways we are only just starting to learn about. Plants have an underground web of data that flows through roots, spores, and the earth. As a plant empath, you can connect to this communication flow and can know what is happening quite some distance away when you develop this skill.

Animal Empaths

Spend time tuning into the animals you are lucky enough to have around you. If you have none of your own, find some friends who have pets. Drop into animal energy fields with your awareness and see what you find there. Spending quiet, calm time getting to know an animal and tuning into it will render some interesting results. Again, keep notes. See if you can match the information you pick up with what is actually going on in that animal's life.

Take an animal communication course and read up on what science can tell you about each animal type. Try connecting with different and unusual animals. Always be safe because any wild animal is not required to keep you safe, and some can be quite dangerous to you no matter how much of a psychic animal empath you are.

Consider volunteering in an animal rescue or shelter and working with animals who need a kind and helpful human to intercede for them. Yes this may be hard for you as you may feel the animal's fear, but it will also help a lot of confused and scared animals find some peace. Helping animals is part of why you have your animal empath ability. As with all empaths, we can benefit the greater good and ease the overall load of pain and suffering in others.

Geomantic Empaths

You need to get barefoot on the earth and regularly dunk yourself in lakes and rivers, too, if at all possible. Go hiking, walking, foraging, and exploring in your local area, and find a few spots that feel right for you. These will be where you go for some much-needed respite.

Consider learning how to dowse. Using a metal or wooden rod as a channel, you can learn to feel into the earth's energies. There are many ways to do so, but simply walking the earth and feeling what it tells you in each spot is a good start. Champion earth clean up and anti-pollution drives as well. You may want to get involved in climate change awareness efforts, as some of these programs may speak directly to your soul.

Precognitive, Emotive, and Dream Empaths

Meditate on what time means to you. Dip into the current of past, present, and future and see if you can energetically link into what they reveal. Take a trip to an antique shop, and if you are allowed, touch a few items to discover what you can "see." Just be sure to do an energetic cleansing of yourself afterwards (we will describe how to do this later in the book).

If you are a telepathic, intuitive, or emotive empath, with permission, work with others and see what you can pick up from them. Let friends or family relate back to you how accurate, or not, you are.

For dream empaths, start by working with your own dreams and make efforts to recall what you dream. Explore methods of lucid dreaming. There are some herbs, like mugwort and blue lotus, that can help with this. Keep a notebook by your bed at all times, and potentially wake yourself during REM sleep to help you better recall your dreams. If you sleep beside someone, see if you are able to connect to their dreams, with their permission, and discuss what you find with them.

Be aware that any exploration into your psychic abilities does come with some dangers to you, so before you start on the journey, it is best to learn how to protect and cleanse your aura and energies. We will get to how to do this in future chapters.

Chapter 4:

Myths and Mysteries

Myths which are believed in tend to become true. –George Orwell

It's likely that you have heard some rather insidious myths and preconceived ideas about empaths held by a bunch of people who really have no clue what they are talking about.

Some of these commonly held ideas can really make you doubt yourself, your sanity, and your reality. People have told me that my sensitivity makes me weak and somehow damaged. Their words have hurt me in the past, but I now know that their thinking is simply a cognitive bias, a faulty thinking loop that simply serves to make themselves feel better. They may have demoralized and undermined me at the time, but now I can let their words go and almost feel bad for them, knowing that they feel empty and sad inside.

There is a rather insidious stereotype of an empath, especially a psychic empath, as being a person who is:

- Pretending to be something they are not

- Using the label of "empath" to make themselves seem special or important

- Dysfunctional and unable to regulate themselves emotionally or in life

Thin-skinned, over-sensitive, fussy, feeble, fragile, weak, temperamental, moody, and overly dramatic

- Co-dependent, perhaps mentally disordered

These painful stereotypes are used to disqualify and undermine the millions of people who are functional empaths. I know many empaths who are nothing like the above profile. For sure, there may be individuals claiming to be empaths who are, in fact, just wanting to use the label to brag or sound special, but this does not mean that their behavior is what you can expect of actual empaths. Quite the contrary.

No two empaths will be exactly the same. Many go about their business never discussing their gifts or even asking for any kind of understanding or help (which, by the way, is not a great idea).

Behind all empath stereotypes lurks a lot of fear. People will naturally fear the unknown and what they don't understand. Empaths don't carry around specific accreditations and qualifications, so there is less science supporting us, and some people will try to discredit, undermine, disqualify, or disprove the very notion of an empath. People sometimes filter what they don't want to admit and only give credence to what helps them prove their opinion. Some folks are also scared of the unknown, and empaths can sometimes be generally lumped in with the supernatural.

Sadly, not everyone is mature or conscious enough to try to truly understand a highly attuned empath. Of course, just because a personality trait seems incomprehensible, almost magical, does not mean that it does not exist. Try not to listen to the doubters and their unkind words.

Common Myths About Empaths

Here are a few of the common unhelpful myths out there, which might be making you doubt yourself.

Myth # 1: You Are Weak and "Soft"

Empaths are some of the strongest people I know. We have to withstand a tangled chaos of emotions and heavy energies bombarding us 24-7, almost from birth, at a level that "normal" people have absolutely no idea about. This can wear us down and weaken our resilience, for sure, but there needs to be a core of strength there, built over a long period of time.

Yes, we are tuned in to the emotional energy around us. Yes, if we don't have our barriers up and protections in place, then we can pick up on all the emotions around us and get confused about what belongs to us and what belongs to others. Until we learn this, to outside eyes, it can look like we are fragile. But we are not.

Myth # 2: You Are Damaged

Trauma can be a part of life, unfortunately. Quite often it has taken one or more toxic people to set off our abilities as a survival response. To stay safe, we developed our extra senses way more than many people ever needed to do. We likely have some work to do on ourselves, but our past trauma is not who we are. Also, not every empath has had a hard childhood. Some people are just born psychic empaths, with their natural abilities already developed.

There are billions of people who have experienced and are experiencing trauma. Helping some of them is one of the reasons you are here- if you wish. Most people avoid, suppress, or ignore their shadow side. A shadow side is the part of ourselves we may think of as "unacceptable"- perhaps a part of us that feels sad or that we feel society will disapprove of. Empaths tend to be more in tune with shadow and engage with it.

Myth # 3: You Are Too Sensitive

It is our sensitivity that makes us empaths, but we can dial this back and learn to manage and control it. It is our extra well-developed senses that form a major part of us. Until we learn to manage our empathic nature, it can seem that we are overly sensitive.

It takes an incredible amount of self-control to not show how what we are sensing affects us. Some empaths shut down completely and may even numb out with alcohol or drugs, and others remain with their senses laid bare like naked, stripped nerves. We are often so busy focusing on just surviving and coping with our own natures that we do not have the spare energy to devote to self care. It can seem like we are overly reactive, but being sensitive can be a good thing, and a mature empath will be able to manage their thoughts, feelings, and energies- they will be far less changeable and reactive to outside stimuli.

Empaths, inadvertently, tend to live under constant pressure from people around them. The fact that most empaths have to survive under such pressure is actually a testimony to our strength and resilience.

Myth # 4: All Empaths Are Introverts

Some empaths are happily able to mix and mingle and are developed and mature enough in their protections and boundaries that the thought of others barely bothers them.

Once we get control of ourselves and our abilities, we may even enjoy socializing and seek it out. If we start following our purpose and helping others—be it animals, people, or the earth itself— we can even begin looking forward to being around those whose energies we feel good with and shielding ourselves when we work with those who need our help. We may still need some quiet time to recharge, but we are fully able to cope with and enjoy the social scene.

Myth # 5: You Are Unable to Succeed at Life

Like with anything and any type of person, there are many variants to a theme. Our nature, being unmanaged and undeveloped, can be quite limiting in that everything feels so raw and intense. This can break us down to some extent, but if we are able to get this under control, we can be incredibly successful in life.

Imagine being able to pick up on bad intentions and on what people are truly thinking. Or picture knowing what energies and resources might exist in the ground under our feet. Clairsentients can tell what has happened before- the history of a place or item. All of this is extremely useful knowledge that can enrich our lives.

Myth # 6: Empaths Are Always Creative

Creativity is a skill that needs to be developed. Maybe you are creative or maybe you're more practical and rational. Just because you can sense others' feelings does not mean that you will be particularly creative. That is up to you.

Myth # 7: You Are Inclined to Be Moody, Anxious, or Depressed

An unprotected empath will get tired, and when you are tired, everything gets harder. When you are picking up on too much information that feels overwhelming, you can stay stuck in a stress cycle, where stress chemicals release into your system and stay there much longer than they should. This hardwires your brain for anxiety, and even panic attacks, if unmanaged.

Also, we empaths learn not to blurt out what we pick up on. We tend to watch what we say and overly control and suppress it. We may not express what we need to out of fear, and that can lead to some depression. Unmanaged thoughts and feelings also complicate the mix.

But really, you are no more moody, anxious, or depressed than any other person, and we all need to learn how to cope with this side of life.

Myth # 8: You Are Lazy

This is a weird one. It may have something to do with the stereotype of a person who is too sensitive. Perhaps people think you're retreating from reality and don't want to interact with life.

This can certainly be true of some people. But again, not a set of qualities particularly tied to being an empath.

It is true that our stress levels sit at a consistently higher level than for others, and this definitely has an impact on our brains and bodies. It can tire us out and can result in illnesses like chronic fatigue, insomnia, and autoimmune disorders if left unmanaged. People might equate these illnesses with laziness, and that's very unfair.

Myth # 9: You Are Self-Absorbed

Empaths are often in service to others and are not generally self-centered or ego-motivated. Souls in service to self are not even in the same league as an empath.

You may at times need to withdraw from emotionally overwhelming situations for your own protection. Preserving your mental and emotional space and health is paramount when you are potentially going to be badly impacted by what is around you.

You may appear inexplicably quiet and moody from the outside. This is often because you are busy processing a load of emotional data. In these moments, self-care and a little TLC are what is needed way more than harsh criticisms and judgments.

Myth # 10: You Have a Personality Disorder

It is easy for someone to try to undermine your entire character by laying it at the feet of a personality disorder. We all sit somewhere on the empath spectrum, and we all have various unresolved issues. It is an "and" situation—you may have a mental health issue, such as anxiety or depression, and be an empath, but one does not cause the other.

Unmanaged empath abilities can exacerbate cognitive disorders, but these would likely exist separately and independently of the empathy bit in any case.

Empaths can find themselves attracting a lot of damaged individuals, who dump their negative energies into our laps. We may have difficulty separating ourselves from this, but again this is a skill you can learn. It's part of self-protection.

Myth # 11: There Is No Such Thing as an Empath

Empaths are highly sensitive to the feelings and emotions of those around them. Science has mixed data on the situation, but that does not mean it is not real or true. There is a lot that science is unable to quantify or comprehend as of now.

Researchers have, however, discovered what they have dubbed "mirror neurons" in the brain, which may help us connect with others' emotions (MacGillivray, 2009). Some people may have more mirror neurons than others, scientifically suggesting that empaths exist.

How do we deal with these unhelpful labels?

- We need to get clear about who we are and what our strengths are, and be actively working on our shadow side.

- We do not need to discuss who we are or what we do with people who have preconceived notions about us.

- We do not need to justify who we are or what we are able to do to anyone.

- We do not need to prove anything to anyone. We simply need to be. Our actions, choices, and the difference we make in the world should, generally, speak for itself to those truly interested in knowing us for real.

It is best not to engage with closed-minded individuals who have already made up their minds. As a psychic empath, your first point of focus should be on your own growth and self-mastery and then, perhaps, on using your strengths to help those you choose to help and who want to be helped.

What that looks like or how it plays out is entirely your own business. If you learn how to find the right kind of people to hang around with, the people who don't break you down and make you feel "less than," but instead build you up and value you, you will find you come up against these ridiculous myths a lot less. Find your tribe and stick with them.

You have a wonderful gift. You just need to learn how to use it safely.

Chapter 5:
The Science Behind Being an Empath

Everything is theoretically impossible, until it is done. –Robert A. Heinlein

Psychic empaths are generally categorized within the spiritual, or alternative, fields. But bearing in mind that these abilities can be developed in most people and that they are easily verifiable and used for many purposes, this level of ability really cuts across the spectrum of life. An empath can be a physicist, a researcher, a therapist, a teacher, or a truck driver. Being an empath is an essential skill that does not have a category or a "side," much like the ability to see, hear, swim, or walk does not have a "side." It just is.

However, because being an empath is lumped in with the supernatural, empaths somehow end up being viewed with disdain and skepticism by those who believe they are scientific and logical. The highly religious- and the highly science-based groups that have attached their personal identity and ego to being one or the other often feel the need to attack this unknown factor. But a true scientist would never lose the opportunity to enquire, discover, and try to comprehend such an interesting thing as empathy. In fact, the growing number of research studies prove that science is very open to understanding the whole range of human ability, including that of the empath. It is a skill that we might be able to develop better in more people once we have a better understanding of it all. That time, I believe, is coming. Only 50 years ago, we would never have believed our current way of life, aided by technology, was even possible, and we may have viewed that with skepticism too. But, here we are.

There is this faulty belief that science and spirituality always need to sit in opposing camps. But that is because science has come to be seen as a group of people, representing specific opinions. In fact, science is merely a method of engaging with the world that requires open-minded inquiry, collection of verifiable data, and the ability to repeat results consistently.

Science and spirituality can co-exist and be on the same team. Why not?

Here is what the researchers have discovered about what it is to be an empath, and some of these results will amaze you.

Mirror Neurons

Mirror neurons, a specialized group of neurons in your brain, dial you into the feelings and thoughts of other people. This connection is also known as emotional contagion. We have mirror neurons that work on physical sensory levels. You can see this at play if you go into a room and start giving off signals of stress or a bad mood. After a few minutes, the whole room may very well be emulating you, unconsciously. You can do this with a good mood, too, by the way, which is probably more altruistic. You can also see mirror neurons at work when you smile and someone smiles back without thinking or when you yawn when somebody else does.

Some people feel this more than others. If someone you are connected to or care about gets hurt, you feel it too. They start crying, and then so do you. They laugh, and you join in without even knowing the joke. Someone gets physically wounded, and you cringe and "feel" the pain. Most people's natural tendency is to reach out and help.

Even in very small children only a few weeks old, researchers see this behavior. Observing this behavior is obviously limited by the infant's inability to speak or move that much, but their responses to their mother dropping an item or hurting herself are very noticeable. If they could get up and help, they would (Simpson et al., 2014). Cute, right?

Mirror neurons are not the only cause of empathy, but they definitely promote empathy for others in most functional brains. In psychic empaths, these mirror-neuron functions are probably a little more developed, and there are fewer natural barriers that help you define the difference between yourself and others.

When you dissolve certain cognitive barriers between you and another person you can literally experience the other in your own mind, emotionally and even physically. Research into mirror neurons shows how people with phantom limbs that watch someone else being touched feel it in their missing limb as if it is real for them (Ramachandran, 2013). In fact, when people experience pain in a phantom limb, they can also experience relief if someone massages that corresponding limb on their separate body. Amazing!

This is also seen with mirror-touch synesthesia, where certain individuals feel the touch sensation when they see others touched, but it has become a disorder because they cannot delineate between touch on someone else and touch on them. You can imagine that this could cause some problems, not knowing where you end and another person begins. For example, unless they can gain control of this disorder, these individuals cannot be surgeons.

Now, it does not take a big leap to extend the idea of mirror neurons into the psychic realm.

Take this one step further. Imagine not being able to put up any barriers and being forced to feel the psychic energy, emotions, or physical sensations of people around you. That is literally what is happening to an untrained psychic empath. No wonder at first we believe we might be going insane.

Electromagnetic Fields

Our entire body generates electromagnetic fields. These actively transmit data about our thoughts and emotions, among other things. Empaths may be particularly good at picking up on that data from others. Often empaths have stronger reactions to electromagnetic changes in the earth and solar bodies like the moon and sun (Orloff, 2018). Geomantic empaths know all about this, I am sure, as they feel this the most.

Dopamine Sensitivity

Research has found that empaths have a higher sensitivity to dopamine, which is a key neurotransmitter that deals with pleasure, mood, and motivation (Orloff, 2018). What this means in real terms is that we need less of this brain chemical to feel rewarded, happy, and pleased. Dopamine sensitivity is also linked to us connecting to another's feelings, which is hardwired into us anyway.

Our connection to others is strongly enhanced by our empathic neural system that is very responsive to the neurotransmitter. This dopamine sensitivity rewards us for simply being an empath and naturally encourages that skill (Orloff, 2018).

In various studies into the brain and social behavior, the empath (or altruist) has shown up as the direct opposite to the psychopathic type of person. In fact, psychopathic brains are virtually unable to recognize emotions in others at all, and their amygdalae are about 18% smaller than usual. In strong empaths, we see the exact opposite, whereas most people sit somewhere in the middle (Milstead, 2018).

There is no getting away from the fact that human beings are social creatures. For some, the ability to dial into various socially geared brain and body systems is stronger. While this is still being researched and is not as yet fully understood, science does agree that psychic empathy is a very real possibility. In fact, they are saying they believe around 2% of the population might be experiencing this (Ewens, 2018). Empaths do scientifically exist.

We, as psychic empaths, definitely already know that, even if those who have not directly experienced this condition may dismiss it as nonsense. Science is definitely inquiring into what it means to be an empath and has been for some time already. As their investigative methods improve, so do the findings on the subject.

Chapter 6:
All the Clairs Explained

Intuition goes before you, showing you the way. Emotion follows behind, to let you know when you go astray. Listen to your inner voice. It is the calling of your spiritual GPS system seeking to keep you on track towards your true destiny. —Anthon St. Maarten

If we take the word back to its Latin roots, *clair* means clear. Over the centuries, people have displayed psychic abilities on multiple levels, so the clair- categories were developed to try and explain what we were dealing with.

A psychic's clair senses are often in alignment with their dominant, more mainstream senses.

Practical Exercise: What Clair Could You Be?

If you are unsure what type of psychic ability you may have, there are some easy ways to find out which one to focus on:

1. Observe yourself when you are talking and describing something. Do you mainly describe using feeling, seeing, auditory, tactile, or taste-linked words? How you learn in terms of descriptive words will tell you a lot here. For example, you might say, "Do you see what I'm saying," or "We can see XYZ," or you might talk more along the lines of "I feel that" or "I hear you."

2. What senses do you feel more drawn towards? Do you listen to a lot of music, or do you prefer looking at pleasing images? Do you find how fabrics and surfaces feel to the touch is one of your fascinations? The senses you use and that impact you the most may very well align to your extrasensory abilities too.

Once you have decided which senses are more "yours," you can then start exploring the linked clair- ability.

Clair- Abilities Defined

Clairvoyance

Clairvoyance is the most visual psychic ability. This is the ability to link into other vibrational frequencies and visually perceive "with the mind's eye" something present in that frequency. A clairvoyant receives extrasensory images, impressions, and symbols in the form of mental pictures perceived without using the physical eyes and beyond the natural limitations of ordinary space and time. These can be visions, dreams, images, or mental movies.

These impressions are easier to perceive in an alpha brain state and while meditating, though many clairvoyants can acquire visual information regarding the past, present, and future in a variety of ways.

To develop clairvoyance start training your brain to observe:

- Look at the world upside down or in a different way.
- On entering a new space, observe all you can about it.
- Try observing something new in a familiar place.

Claircognizance

Claircognizance is a clear knowing. You suddenly just know something you could not have known in any natural way. You did not hear it or see it. It can happen as a sudden download or flash of insight. Some people talk about gut intuition, or instincts, and these abilities may well be interlinked.

To develop this:

- Raise your energetic vibrations–we speak about this in Chapter 7.

- Open yourself to the downloads safely, from time to time, to see what you might pick up. Time will prove you right or wrong.

Clairintellect

Clairintellect is a fascinating ability indeed. Very close in nature to claircognizance, it is slightly different in that this sense is often linked to specific intellectual pursuits, like mathematics or writing. The person does know how they got to the answers and may not even be able to reproduce the action or show their workings. They just got the answer or the information, and there it is. This can be seen in some forms of channeling.

To develop this skill:

- Practice automatic writing. Sit and channel whatever comes to you.

- Get into a flow state when you use your everyday skills and talents where you are not consciously controlling any outcomes but just fully immersed in the moment.

Clairaudience

Clairaudience is the perception of sounds and words from sources broadcast from the spiritual realm. It can also be mental tones, which are perceived without the aid of the physical ear and beyond normal time and space constraints. The tones and vibrations are more easily perceived during an alpha state and during meditation although clairaudients can receive verbal and sound-related information wherever they are. The majority of channelers (also known as mediums) work with both clairvoyance and clairaudience.

To develop this skill

- It is possible to uplift yourself through the power of sound frequencies. Through our sense of hearing, we can find a whole soundscape of meditative frequencies that can empower and connect us more strongly with our spiritual element. We can then use this spiritually infused strength to improve our external environment. These frequencies are often used therapeutically with ambient sounds to induce calm. Not only does sound affect our ears, it also affects us on a molecular and energetic level. For example, 525 Hz music reduces stress. and psychic awakening is encouraged using the 432 MHz frequency

- Listen in with your empath senses rather than just your ears. Beyond words you hear, listen for what you can pick up from the tone of voice of a speaker.

- Use music therapy, sound healing, and sound energy modalities like Tibetan singing bowls, tuning forks, and chimes.

Clairsentience

Clairsentience (clear sensation) is the ability to understand information through a "feeling" within the entire body without any external stimuli.

Pretty much any of the development ideas for the other clair senses will work to develop this, as it is a pretty all-encompassing skill.

To develop this skill in general

- Use meditation and reflection regularly.
- Tune in to your senses and try some sensory exercises like deep listening, focusing on tastes, textures, smells, and sight. Do it one sense at a time if you can and fully immerse yourself in this way.

Clairsalience

Clairscent or clairsalience is a clear sense of smell. It is to smell a fragrance or odor of a substance or food that is not in one's immediate surroundings. A person can perceive these odors without the aid of a physical nose and beyond the confines of normal time and space.

To develop this skill:

- Spend time every day smelling your environment—flowers, food, spices, natural body odors, animals, plants, earth, and even water. Take yourself on a scent journey.
- See if you can pick up on a person's emotional or physical state through smelling their natural body odor.
- See what memories you can connect to by smelling various scents.

Clairtangency

Psychometry is more commonly known as clairtangency (clear touching). Handling an object or touching an area and receiving information previously unknown to the clairtangent about the object or its owner. This is often experienced when you shake hands or hold a personal item belonging to someone else.

To develop this skill

- Ask others if you may hold their hand while you see what you can sense. Ask them how accurate you may be.
- Take a trip to an antique shop and handle a few of the items.
- Take a nature walk and touch the trees and rocks along the way.

Clairgustance

Clairgustance (clear tasting) is sensing through taste. It is to taste a substance without putting anything in one's mouth. Through taste, those who possess this ability are said to be able to perceive the essence of substances from the spiritual or ethereal realms.

To develop this skill

- Immerse yourself in the food you eat and the liquids you drink. Make it a sensory experience where you drop your awareness fully into the moment and the experience.
- Take a taste adventure at a food market or restaurant by trying out various tastes you normally wouldn't.
- Focus on taste sensations by sampling a range of foods, herbs, and spices in your kitchen.

Clairempathy

Clairempathy (clear emotion) refers to the ability to psychically tune in to the emotional experience of a person, place, or animal. Clairempathy is a sort of telepathy, or sense to feel within one's self- the attitude, illness, or emotion of another person or entity. This skill can be developed by using all the exercises given to you in this book.

You may not have strong psychic senses right at this moment, but with patience and time you can develop and strengthen them. It is always a good idea to first learn some psychic protection and hygiene first, though.

Keep a journal, and record all your experiments and exercises as you go. Learning mindfulness techniques and how to observe yourself and your environment are a very good start.

Chapter 7:
Psychic Protection

He who creates a poison also has the cure. He who creates a virus also has the antidote. He who creates chaos also has the ability to create peace. He who sparks hate also has the ability to transform it to love. He who creates misery also has the ability to destroy it with kindness. He who creates sadness also has the ability to convert it to happiness. He who creates darkness can also be awakened to produce illumination. He who spreads fear can also be shaken to spread comfort. Any problems created by the left hand of man can also be solved with the right for he who manifests anything also has the ability to destroy it. —Suzy Kassem

Once you realize that you are an empath, the very next vital step is to start putting up a barrier between you and the excess emotions and information out there that you don't want to feel.

This will mean that once you get stronger and better at doing this, with enough practice, you will no longer have to fear being an empath. You will be able to move through crowds, touch things, and even enter toxic energy areas and emerge unscathed by them.

It will mean the most incredible sense of peace, maybe even a level of calm you have never experienced before. And that's really something if you have been struggling along unprotected for a while. We will cover what to do with any excess energy you have absorbed in the next chapter, but for now, let's learn how to make ourselves safer.

Boundaries

Setting boundaries is a basic life skill that many people do not fully understand and an area that many empaths struggle with.

Here's the thing: You have this one life, perhaps more, but we can't know for sure. So let's go with that for now. Every person gets their own life, right? It's not very long. Only around 25,000 days (or 900 months) if you live an average lifespan.

The idea is that each of us get to decide how to spend that time. It's really intrusive and obstructive for any one of us to try and take over anyone else's life without permission. But that is basically what is happening when someone crosses your boundaries. They are taking their agenda and imposing it on you. There is something they want, and they want a piece of your time and energy to do it.

Now, I'm not saying that everyone does this consciously or with bad intentions. In fact, most people don't set out to steamroll right over your boundaries. Many of your boundaries are specific to you and people don't always guess what they are. There are obvious, more universal boundaries like 'do no harm' or 'don't steal someone's property.' But there are many specifics that you personally want or don't want, like or don't like.

Here is what you need to know:

- Having everyday boundaries is the first step to being able to create psychic boundaries.

- Boundaries are something you have to actively put in place yourself. You cannot expect anyone to do this for you, except perhaps your parents when you are little.

- You do need to have boundaries. These are the limits within which you feel safe and happy to operate. Anything outside these limits will leave you feeling unsafe and unhappy.

- Remember not to disrespect someone else's boundaries while trying to maintain your own.

You first of all need to decide what your boundaries are.

Practical Exercise: What Are My Boundaries?

With pen and paper in hand take some time to think about

1. What words, actions, and situations do you not like? What situations make you feel uncomfortable or stressed out? Think back to past experiences to help with this.

2. What was it about the words/action/situation that you did not like?

3. What value of yours do you think wasn't being respected?

4. Where in your life are you letting people cross this boundary? What are they doing and when?

5. What would you want them to do or say instead?

Some examples of boundaries may be:

- Do not disrespect my time.

- Keep at least one meter away from me, outside my personal space bubble, and do not touch me without my permission.

- Don't touch my stuff without my permission.
- Do not use hurtful words to me or around me.
- Do not phone me after 8 p.m. or before 7 a.m.
- Do not interrupt me when it is my turn to speak.
- Do not devalue my career /eating habits/ choice of partner

You can make your list of boundaries as long or as short as you wish. Just make sure the list describes the things that are an absolute no go for you, at the bare minimum.

Next, you need to make sure that the significant people in your life know what your boundaries are. You don't need to be harsh or abrasive about communicating your boundaries with people in your life- just tell them when appropriate. Most reasonable, functional people will do their best to cooperate. If they forget, you can gently remind them. If people persist in not respecting what you are requiring, you can consider putting systems in place that work independently of their selfish behavior.

For example, say your mother keeps calling after 9 p.m. at night and you go to bed at 8:30 p.m. You could say, "Mom, I go to bed (or watch my movies/read) after 8 p.m. and will not be available for calls after this time in future. Please only call (or text) after 8pm if it is a real emergency."

By doing this, you have politely and clearly communicated what you need. If she persists in calling, you can silence your phone and simply not take calls. Or silence your phone and only reply to emergency texts. Or find another close family member who can follow your rules and add them as an emergency contact so that their calls go through even when your phone is on sleep mode.

If you have a tough time saying no, start small. Practice saying it to yourself in the mirror. Graduate to saying no to small, insignificant requests from other people. Your confidence will grow. Practice saying no and not giving any reason for it. It may feel uncomfortable, but stick with it. Over time your discomfort lessens, and you feel more empowered. You will be able to say no about the bigger stuff eventually.

Also, bear in mind that, especially with toxic people, when you put a boundary in place, there will be pushback. Extremely toxic people may even throw a tantrum or try to punish you in some way. This is an even more important time when to stay strong and stick with enforcing your boundary. If you give in now, you are only making it worse for yourself in the long run by teaching people that if they push hard enough, they will always get what they want. Sticking with your boundaries will eventually pay off. The noise and pushback will die down, and people will acclimatize to the new normal. For me setting boundaries with my family was one of the hardest things I had to learn to do, but it was oh so worth it to get my time and mental energy back. Ultimately, for a small period of pain, you are buying yourself a world of peace and freedom.

Energy

Once you've established your everyday boundaries, you can start putting psychic boundaries in place.

Psychic boundaries have a lot to do with how we work with energy. As discussed earlier in the book, our bodies generate an electromagnetic field. Our body also has energy pathways that approximate to the channels of our nervous system. Acupuncturists have been using this knowledge for thousands of years already.

The energy field our body gives off extend quite some distance from us, and this is what some of us are able to see (or empathically connect into) as an aura. Often, when we read a person's physical or emotional health state, this means that our energy (our aura) is interacting with theirs and downloading information that way. That is not the only way we download information, but it is one of the main ways we pick up on data that we couldn't have otherwise known. Auric fields contain all sorts of data, such as our thoughts, emotions, memories, physical health, intentions and even impending illnesses and diseases that haven't taken hold yet.

Our aura exists in layers or etheric fields Below are the 7 layers that make up our auras:

1. The etheric aura layer runs close to the body, extending out about two to four inches. Some people see this layer as a faint violet-gray mist which connects to the base chakra.

2. The emotional layer extends about an inch or three outside of the etheric layer, connects to the sacral chakra, and shows our emotions.

3. The mental layer extends about three to eight inches out and connects to the solar plexus chakra. It is often seen as yellow.

4. The astral layer extends out about one foot or so and has a rainbow color. It is where we connect to others, form energetic cords, and connect from our physical body into our spirit and that of others. It is often a rosy pink color and connects to the heart chakra.

5. The etheric template layer extends out about two feet, connects to the throat chakra and is a blueprint of the

physical body. Illness and disease can easily be seen in this layer.

6. The celestial layer extends out up to two-and-a-half feet and connects to the third-eye chakra. This energy layer is to do with intuition and enlightenment. Some people describe the color as mother of pearl.

7. The ketheric layer can extend up to three feet outside the body. It connects to the crown chakra and may be seen as a white or golden light. It holds soul information, including past and future lifetimes.

You can teach yourself to see auras in a number of ways. One way is to look indirectly at a person—as if your eyes are glancing just off their edges a little bit. You can do this with anyone, as well as with plants and animals.

An easy way to practice seeing auras at any time is to begin with your own hand against a pale or white background. Keep looking at your hand and eventually you will see some colors that are not simply the shadows and shapes caused by the afterimages on your retina of what you were previously looking at.

Another way to feel into your own energy field is to hold your hands together, and then slowly move them apart. At a certain point you will feel some static, or tingling, and that is a good indication that you are feeling the edge of your physical aura layers.

I have briefly mentioned chakras, which is a Sanskrit word for "wheel." Our chakras are energy centers that align with major organs or bundles of nerves in our bodies.

There are seven main chakras running down the centerline of our bodies:

1. Our root chakra sits at the end of our tailbone, and it is all about stability, our physical identity, and being grounded. When the root chakra is open and aligned, we feel secure emotionally and physically. This chakra's color is red.

2. Our sacral chakra is just below the belly button, is orange in color, and deals with our sexual and creative elements.

3. Our solar plexus chakra sits in our upper abdomen, is a yellow color, and governs self-esteem and confidence.

4. The heart chakra sits at the center of the chest near the heart, is green in color, and relates to love and compassion. It bridges the gap between our lower physical energy layers and our higher spiritual energy fields. This chakra is most often blocked in untrained empaths because we tend to put others' needs before our own, to our own detriment. It will stay blocked until we get better at boundary control.

5. The throat chakra is blue and relates to all matters of communication.

6. The third-eye chakra sits between and just above your eyes. It is purple (indigo) and relates to your ability to see clearly on a psychic level as well as intuition and imagination.

7. Your crown chakra sits at the very top of your head, is a violet or white color, and relates to awareness, intelligence, and your connection to source or a higher power/energy.

You don't need to know too much about auras and chakras right now, just that they are there and can indicate certain states to those who can work with them. As you develop your energetic healing and awareness abilities, you will be able to see auric colors, or feel their energy, more easily. This will help give you direct information about yourself and others and serve as an early warning system when a highly toxic person approaches.

We will speak more about how to start working with your own auric field and chakra centers in the self-care chapter. You really want to keep your energy unclogged, free-flowing, and aligned. This is what will help you feel good on every level, including psychically.

The main rules for managing your energy include:

- Regular grounding practices
- Cleansing your chakras and aura
- Knowing how to draw in your energy field and protect your energy
- Knowing the feel of your energy versus someone or something else
- Asking for help when you feel out of your depth or overwhelmed

Psychic Protection

Protection is not about living in fear. Since, as an empath, your energy is more open and sensitive, we just want to make sure you can dial down the noise when you need to. When you're protected your abilities are more about choice and less about stress. You choose when you want to use your gifts rather than having them overwhelm you.

Because we are mainly linking into others, and the world, energetically, it is on this level that we will need our strongest protections as an empath. There are loads of ways to put protections in place- I am going to take you through quite a few, and then it is up to you to choose the ones that work best. However, whatever you do, you absolutely must make a daily protection practice part of your routine.

Our goals are to:

- Get control of our own thoughts, emotions, and shadow side
- Clear our own energies regularly
- Let go of things that no longer serve us
- Cut off unwanted cords and attachments
- Put certain barriers and psychic boundaries in place every day

We need to protect ourselves from other people's moods and thoughts, unwanted energetic cords, psychic vampires and attacks, and everyday stresses and strains. Just like we put sunscreen on, so we must put psychic protection in place. So how do we do this?

Powerful Exercise: Know Your Own Energy

Spend some quiet time with yourself, on a day where you are well rested, without any new, exciting, or stressful events happening (if that is possible). Then:

1. Take a brisk walk or do about 15 minutes of any form of exercise or movement that appeals to you. Have a light snack if you're hungry and drink a glass of water. This is to ensure that no physical needs or stress chemicals interfere with this work.

2. Do an energetic cleansing and grounding practice (see the next chapter for how to do so).

3. Do some meditation or yoga- whatever works best for you to relax and be calm. If you're not already a practitioner of meditation or yoga, sitting comfortably and breathing deeply with your eyes closed will also work. After a few minutes of whichever of the above practices you've chosen, start observing yourself.

   a. What does it feel like to be you?

   b. Can you feel into your energy and energy level? Ask yourself:

      - Is your energy high, low, or just purring along?
      - Is it brittle or stretchy?
      - Is it firm or pliant?
      - Is it round, square, triangular, or shapeless?
      - What color does it feel like? Try to visualize it.
      - What does it "smell" like"?

4. Stay sitting and observing your energy for as long as you can comfortably do so. Check in with it fully every few minutes to see if it has changed in any way.

5. Once finished, journal or make a note of what you noticed.

6. Do this same exercise at least twice a week over about a month to get a baseline on yourself and also to teach yourself what "you" feel like.

7. Also feel into your energy in a range of different situations- but not when you are interacting with others.

This will give you a very good sense of what your own energy feels like. It is important to know your own baseline in order to help differentiate between you and others. Practicing this exercise really helps you know when you might have taken on someone else's energy.

Visualization

Visualization is a big part of psychic protection and very simple to do. Nothing is required other than your mind and imagination. This is all about will, intent, and energy focus.

There are two main ways to visualize your energetic protection.

One way is to imagine a great bubble of shining white light surrounding you, your car, your home, and even your workspace, like an energy force field. You can also make the color of this bubble silver if you are concerned about any particularly negative energies seeking you out. Evil does not like its own reflection.

Other visualizations you can try include picturing a suit of armor around you, or symbols of protection (like the pentagram, seeing eye, or ankh) or whatever symbolizes safety and protection to you.

Visualization protection can be done once a day or whenever you feel you are going into a potentially bad or energetically noisy environment.

Other visualizations to try include:

- Imagining your aura, and then seeing it pull in tight, dense, and close to your body, surrounding you
- Taking your hand and "zipping" up your energy from your lowest chakra to the crown chakra. Do this slowly and with the intent to shut down and out the outside world

The general white or silver light protection is fine to create and leave in place, but the last two visualizations mentioned should be reversed once you are in a safe space. You don't want to shut out life all the time. To reverse these last two visualizations:

- Imagine your aura relaxing and gently wafting or spilling outward, almost like releasing the tight string from around a tied up Christmas tree.

- Take your hand and "unzip" your energy from your crown chakra to the lowest chakra. Do this slowly and with the intent to expand your energy into the outside world

Using protective visualizations are a two-way street- they will make it harder for others to read or communicate with you, and these visualizations will also protect you from picking up on information from others as you remain energetically safe within yourself. Just make sure to sometimes reverse the protective visualizations or you can start feeling a bit like you're in solitary confinement if you are not careful.

A certain amount of energetic interaction is needed with the world to learn, grow, and keep your energy flowing in a healthy way. You can choose where and when to let your energy be free and unprotected. For some time, I would only let my energy mingle with the world when out in nature, on my own or with my dogs. Now I feel so much stronger than I used to, and I only protect my energy in the ways above when I know I will be encountering a lot of energy I don't want to take on. I still visualize a comforting white or silver light around me every morning when I wake up- that exercise is consistently helpful to me.

Protective Tools

Feel free to use tools and supporting aids if you feel you need them. The below types of tools are particularly useful in the beginning, but you will probably find that the stronger you get, the less necessary they really are.

There are a load of options you can use to help support your protective efforts.

Crystals like black tourmaline, obsidian, sodalite, amethyst, and lapis lazuli are all helpful. If you decide to use crystals, learn how to work with them. They, too, need cleansing and charging. Here are a few ways to cleanse and charge your crystals:

- Keep your crystals together with a piece of selenite
- Run them under water for about a minute each
- Burn some sage, preferably outdoors, and for 30 seconds to a minute hold your crystal in the smoke.
- Use chanting, singing bowls, or a tuning fork. Sound healing will cleanse multiple crystals at once.
- Leave them out in the sunshine or moonlight for a few hours to clear and recharge them.
- Don't let other people touch them, and if they do, recleanse them.

You can wear your protective stones as jewelry, carry them in a pouch or pocket, or use them in a crystal grid or pattern (at the points of whatever symbol you like, or just at the four quarters), in a room or for an entire property.

Talismans and amulets, like the Eye of Horus, pentacle, ankh, cross, or any symbol that holds protective meaning for you, can be used as jewelry or a tattoo or visualized drawn in light over your body or an area.

Prayers, blessings, and meaningful mantras might be options for you to charge up your crystals as well.

Protective Spirits

The animal and plant world contains many allies that will help you if you ask.

Herbs can be used as an incense, oils, tinctures, and essences. For example, yarrow, rosemary, vervain, lavender, eucalyptus, flannel flower, juniper, fringed violet, sage, and tea tree are all strong protectors. I grow rosemary and lavender plants around my home and all through my garden. You can pick and use a sprig, keeping it in a shoe or pocket, as an effective measure of protection as well. Ask the tree or plant spirit for protection while you are at it.

If you are able to energetically connect with your pets, you can ask for their support. Dogs are very connected with their owners and want to reach out and help. They will sense that you need them when you feel down or when you simply ask for assistance. Cats are especially great at filtering out bad energies from you and their surroundings. Their purr alone, which resonates at a specific MHz, is very healing. Do you notice that your pet will often lie on your lap or chest, and you may immediately feel better? Let them aid you. If they can't take the heat, they will also communicate that.

Shamanic practice involves the use of animal spirits and guides. If you cannot find a shamanic healer to work with who can teach you, then you can call on the energy of the animal that most appeals to you.

Lastly, you can appeal to the energy of your home, or your house spirits, for protection. A space can develop a "soul" of sorts, which likes being acknowledged and honored. "Gifting" these spirits by tidying up your home, or lighting candles in a specific spot or altar as an offering to the house spirits is quite a nice gesture, and you may find the energy in your home reacts very well to this.

Practical Exercise: Calling an Animal Spirit Protector

1. Do a thorough space and self cleansing. Use visualization, sound healing, water, or any one of the aforementioned cleansing rituals.

2. It is often better to do this outdoors, if possible.

3. Burn some incense or light a candle and add whatever feels appropriate to create a ritual to honor the spirit you wish to connect with.

4. Ask out loud for your animal spirit to make itself known to you. Don't judge or overthink what comes to you. Your spirit can represent an animal from the everyday world, or from myth, folklore, or legend. My spirit animal is a big friendly Labrador with floppy years, who can magically transform into a Direwolf when I need her to.

5. Sit quietly, meditate, breathe deeply, and wait.

6. See what comes to you. It might be a physical sign, where an actual animal shows itself to you, or you may just get a sense of the animal's energy or see it in your mind's eye. It will feel right and strong.

7. When you connect, greet, and honor the animal spirit. Make an offering to it in your mind, giving it your attention and appreciation. Ask it for its protection over you.

8. You can find or make little statues or pictures of your animal spirit as a reminder that it is there.

Guides, angels, and ascended masters are also options for psychic and spiritual protection. At different points in my life, I have asked different spirits for help. You can decide what you need at any given time.

Practical Exercise: Connect With Your Spirit Guide
The first thing to know is that you don't really need to get your spirit guide's attention. Your spirit guides have always been there, watching and helping you however they can. But you can do certain things so that you are more open to hearing their messages.

- Wear a lapis lazuli stone to open up your channels and know your truth.

- Keep your vibrations high through energetic clearing, visualizing, grounding, diet, and mindset, as this makes it easier for your guides to connect with you.

- Listen to your gut, or that feeling of knowing.

- Visualize that you are walking along a forest path or the beach, or see yourself in a beautiful garden. Wait patiently and see who comes to you. Your spirit guide can take many forms- even that of people you know or once knew.

Develop Your Willpower

Behind most boundaries, mundane or psychic, lies the strength of your will. Willpower links to strength of mind and purpose, and it can be developed just like any muscle. Consider it a mental and spiritual muscle, if you like.

Some ways you can strengthen your willpower include (Dandapani, 2019):

- Always finish things you start. For example, make your bed after you finish sleeping.

- Always try to do a little better than you think you can.

- Do just a little more than you think you can do.

- Look for opportunities to exercise your willpower. The more you successfully do this the stronger you get. For example, choose something constructive over that next series binge, or choose that healthy fruit over that bag of cookies. Each time you choose your path and follow through you prove to your mind that what you say and choose will happen. Then when you say "I am protected" then you are.

It sounds simplistic, yet over time, it builds this strength, which in turn helps you to build better psychic muscles and skills.

Energy Vampires, Narcissists and All the 'Paths

Some people are badly damaged. Their energy is low, they vibrate at a very low level, their emotions are unchecked and unregulated, and they desperately need more energy from wherever they can get it. These people desperately want to feel better, and empaths generate an amazing feel-good vibe that they are drawn to.

Energy vampires can include people with personality disorders, like narcissistic personality disorder, borderline personality disorder, or some other socio-cognitive issue that impacts how they operate in the world. Some energy vampires have no diagnosed personality disorder, but have certain traits that can be extremely draining to empaths nonetheless.

Look for a pattern. People can have a bad day and need some extra support from time to time but that does not make them an energy vampire. A vampire consistently over time leaves you feeling exhausted. They are often easily spotted because they are the very dramatic, overly emotional ones who behave erratically and have loads of faulty thinking behind their words. They have little self-regulation or self-awareness. Intentional energy vampires do not see the problem with taking up your time and energy, even if it damages you in the process. If you resist, they might try guilt trips or mind games to get reconnected or get what they want from you.

One of the biggest issues empaths face is that we attract these toxic individuals to our warm, healing, giving energy. The problem is that certain types cannot be healed or made whole, so they just drain us and leave us and themselves broken at the end. Certain individuals cannot see that their use of us is not helping them or us. They so badly want to feel better, which we can understand on a level. But this situation is a bit like a drowning person pulling you down so you both go under the waves.

It is an empath's nature to want to help, support, and heal. Sometimes this can spring up from slightly selfish motivations. When others are whole and stable around us, they will not impact us as badly, so we also in turn get to feel a bit better. Putting protections in place makes this a moot point. We can feel better regardless, and then we can choose to help others from a place of power rather than necessity.

But back to the energy vampires. There are some people we simply cannot help. The nature of a true narcissist is that they have been damaged fairly early on by some childhood lack or trauma. They seem to freeze emotionally at this point, and so they grow up physically but remain immature emotionally. Picture a toddler who wants everything their way, and you can see what is really going on but they can't. Add to this a lot of fear on their part. Part of the profile of an energy vampire is insecurity and a lot of feelings of self-hatred, buried deep within. That darkness that they carry is extremely scary for them to face, and so they never do. It is beyond their abilities. Because they cannot face their shadows, they have very little chance of ever truly solving these issues or of growing emotionally.

Change is pretty unlikely in these circumstances. At the same time, a narcissist knows what works, what is acceptable, and what is not. Often they are very good at charming, convincing, and persuading when they wish. That can be confusing when they suddenly turn on you and lash out, generally when you have stopped being useful to them or you see what's going on within them and they find out. Add to this the fact that empaths are especially drawn to chaos and pain—often innocently thinking that they can help—and we have a recipe for disaster. In these circumstances, having boundaries, plus psychic and energetic protection are not just vital, they are mandatory. That is if you can't get away from people like this completely.

To be clear, not every selfish or badly behaved person is a narcissist. Some people may have elements of narcissism or sit somewhere on the spectrum closer to the full narcissist, but they may also have the ability to grow and learn, to hear some criticism, and to start objectively evaluating themselves. Don't fall into the trap of labeling everyone a narcissist because then it becomes a "crying wolf" situation, and when a true narcissist comes along, nobody will believe you.

Many energy vampires are actually sending out their draining energy unconsciously. They need healing and help, and they also have no or few boundaries in place. They inadvertently siphon off your energy and that of everyone around them. A very sick child, or even an animal, can inadvertently pull on your energy to support their own, and in these cases, you can choose to actively share what you have, within reason. Giving of your energy becomes an act of choice and will, and you can decide how much and when to shut it down, simply by thinking about it.

There are also conscious energy vampires who sense that your aura and energy is open (as it is if you are an untrained empath), and so it is extremely easy for them to tap into you to supplement themselves.

This all comes back to the fact that you must acknowledge that you cannot save the world and that each soul has their own path to walk. If someone is painfully damaging you, then you need to take steps to protect yourself, and sometimes that might mean cutting them out of your life altogether. If you are in a situation where you feel someone is consciously hurting you with dangerous, toxic energy, there is a lot of material online about how to disconnect, set strong boundaries, and walk away.

Watch out for people who:

- You always feel depleted and drained after being around. Don't focus on what they are saying or doing so much as how it leaves you feeling in the end.

- Leave you feeling inexplicably tired every time they make contact.

- Invade your energy every time they are around. If you know what your base energy is like, and have protections in place, you will notice when someone is trying to tap into you.

- Do not respect any boundaries and take up your time and energy without asking. Being with them always feels invasive and disruptive, or simply overwhelming.

The answer?

You need to disengage, cut energetic cords, and set up your boundaries on every level. Better yet, if possible, don't spend time with or on energy vampires. Don't get sucked into conversations or any other kind of connection that consistently leaves you feeling drained. If you have to talk to these people, keep your conversations neutral and continually refocus them on whatever it is that absolutely must be discussed. Ignore any other complaints or negativity- simply don't answer it, respond to it, or acknowledge it in any way. Then you avoid being pulled into the game.

Nobody gets to feed off you. As a psychic empath, when you grow better at working with energy, you will realize that you get to choose what energy you share with others. Your energy is not finite. A trained empath knows how to quickly recharge with psychic self-care, so energy vampires are much less of a problem.

Allowing these one-sided relationships to persist will result in you getting physically, emotionally, and psychically ill and out of balance. If you are in this situation, please get some help and put protections in place sooner rather than later.

Chapter 8:
Psychic Self-Care

If you celebrate your differentness, the world will, too. It believes exactly what you tell it—through the words you use to describe yourself, the actions you take to care for yourself, and the choices you make to express yourself. Tell the world you are a one-of-a-kind creation who came here to experience wonder and spread joy. Expect to be accommodated. —Victoria Moran

If you give it some thought, you may realize that not a lot of good grows out of fear. Sure, fear can motivate some actions, but it is not a great long-term plan. Children raised in fear develop harmful survival mechanisms that can result in people-pleasing, codependency, insecurity and anxiety, narcissism or any number of trauma-based reactions that live with them for the rest of their lives. People who make choices from a base of fear tend to be reactive, thinking from their animal brains. Anger, distrust, insecurity, and anxiety are all part of this picture. Dial any toxic or destructive behavior backwards and it is extremely likely that underneath it all is some kind of fear driving the machinery.

Understanding this is the first step, and then looking inwards to find where fear may be driving your own behavior is a great next step. The opposite of fear is, of course, love. But love does not start somewhere "out there." To be able to channel love and share it with others, you first need to have it inside of you.

If you have not been shown much love, especially by your primary caregivers, it is quite common to think you are not worthy of it and that something is wrong with you. You may simply not know how it is done or how it feels.

If you are filled with self-hatred and have no kindness and compassion for yourself, the odds are that no matter what your best intentions are, your energy will leak out organically onto those around you. So whatever your story is, and whatever you believe you are guilty of or have shame about, you need to work through it, learn from it, and let go so that you can be free and breathe easy in the present moment.

There are a few ways to start healing old wounds:

1. Work with a cognitive-behavioral (CBT) therapist or psychodynamic therapist to face and heal past wounds. This helps you get another perspective on your life and reframe some of your unhelpful inner dialogue.

2. Start showing yourself some love:

    a. Journal every day, listing a few things that you got right that day and one or two things you like about yourself.

    b. Prop a picture of yourself as a little kid up on the bathroom mirror and say the nice, loving things that little kid needs to hear.

    c. Allow for mistakes and reframe how you think about them. Mistakes are really just learning opportunities. While at times it feels bad to make mistakes, you can either take the lessons you've learned and move forward, or you can get stuck in the blame/shame cycle that just breaks you down.

d. Get some perspective on other people's opinions of you. Do they have the whole story? Do they really know what your life is like? Does their opinion really matter? Will they be around in a year, or five? Will they have to live with the consequences of your choices?

The odds are that you are doing your best with what you know and have at hand. Learn to say "so what" to unhelpful feedback and opinions. If it helps, imagine how you would defend a friend who was being subjected to the same kind of opinions or disapproval you have for yourself.

Put some distance between yourself and the negative people who always leave you feeling broken down, "less than," or bad.

Every day do one small act of kindness for yourself.

3. Keep growing and learning. The more you learn about yourself and others and grow as a self-aware, conscious being, the more healing will come your way.

Being the person you needed around for you as a little kid and treating yourself with care, kindness, compassion, and love will strengthen you in ways you maybe can't imagine right now. Just make a start somewhere with this, and keep going. Sooner rather than later you will look back and realize how very far you have come and how much your life has changed for the better with this self-love, self-care approach.

First Sort Out Your Foundations

Basic self-care underlies psychic self-care. If you are tired, hungry, ill, in physical pain, dehydrated, or way too sedentary that will affect your physical health, which will, in turn, affect your brain, mood, and emotions. And all of that will affect your psychic strength and resilience Everything is interlinked.

Take some time to assess your basics:

- How are you eating? Regular healthy meals and snacks are vital to keep your blood sugar levels stable. The sugars in your blood drive your energy levels and sustain life. Whole grains, vegetables, fruits, complex carbohydrates, seeds, nuts, legumes, herbs, and spices are all great for supporting good health. From a psychic point of view, meat does tend to make your energy sluggish and lower your energetic vibrations, making it harder to reach your spirit guides or work actively on a psychic level. But not everyone wants to live vegan. So if you must eat meat, fish, and eggs, stick to leaner meat of animals farmed with kindness and care.

- Avoid highly processed foods, too many additives (which tend to create a chemical storm your body does not know how to deal with), simple carbs, and excess sugars, like sweet sodas, energy bars and sugary cereals. Limit your sweet treats or replace them with healthier options, like frozen yogurt, mashed/frozen berries, and bananas.

- Make sure you are drinking enough healthy liquids. Water, herbal teas, and veggie and fruit juices are all good options. You need about a liter-and-a-half of liquid a day, and it does not need to be all water. Just bear in mind that water is easiest on your system to process.

- Are you moving around enough? Research shows that around 30 minutes of brisk movement every day directly impacts your mood and improves it greatly, to the point that it has been found to be a good replacement to antidepressants (Netz, 2017). Movement helps your body circulate fluids and get rid of toxins, plus it builds muscle strength and physical resilience.

- Gut health helps calm systemic inflammation and helps with mood and overall health. Care for it with probiotics and gut-friendly foods as much as possible.

- How are you sleeping? This is the time when your body rests and your brain detoxes, sorts through the day's memories, and does general housekeeping. Getting a sleep routine in place- getting enough exercise during the day, making sure your sleeping area is calm, quiet, and comfortable, and allowing enough time for quality rest are so important. Also, sleep means dreaming and that is a useful tool for any psychic.

This is not a general health book, and all of the above can be looked into more thoroughly with research and talking to medical or naturopathic professionals. But your physical health cannot be dismissed or overlooked if you want to strengthen and grow in your psychic abilities. Even the Buddha agreed that the physical body requires some care. Asceticism, self-neglect, and deprivation are not the best ways to reach enlightenment.

Basic Psychic Hygiene

Just as you brush your teeth and bathe your body regularly, so you need to cleanse your energetic self. It does not take a lot of skill or effort to do, but it does need to become part of your routine each day for best effect.

Clearing and cleansing your energy is easiest done in these ways:

- **White light visualizations**: When you are in the shower or during your meditations or time outdoors, visualize light pouring down through the top of your head, through your body, and then out through your feet into the earth. Picture all the psychic mud and muck that you may have picked up from people, things, and places washing away. Let the earth process and recycle this as she is so very good at doing. If you like, visualize it burning away in the earth's magma core. Combine this with your daily psychic protection I shared with you earlier in the book.

- **Crystal healing**: You can place crystals the same colors as your chakras on your body, along the corresponding chakra, and lie like that for a while, perhaps meditating to maximize the use of time.

- **Chakra visualization**: You can visualize each energy center or chakra, feel into it energetically, draw energy up from the earth or from the air around you, and pour it into each chakra one by one. Visualize the color of the chakra, and see them spinning and glowing freely.

- **Water immersion**: Getting into water is incredibly soothing and cleansing for the spirit. I love regular dips in the ocean or a local river or lake whenever I can fit it into my schedule and the season is right for it. A bath with herbs or oils such as lemon, lavender, or rosemary, some Epsom salts, and maybe even a crystal or two in the water is like making a big magic cleansing potion you can climb into.

If you feel you need something more, find a local energy worker, reiki practitioner, or someone similar to help you out. But before you allow a stranger to work in your energy field, check in with your intuition and see if they feel safe for you. I am very careful who I allow to work on or with me energetically, and once I find someone who I can trust and who knows what they are doing, I tend to stick with them. Picking up a psychic at a local fair without doing some checks is taking quite a risk.

A last word on protection. We are not only protecting our energy from other people but also from energy entities of all kinds that might be attracted to our psychic nature. As a psychic, the odds are that you are actively experimenting with a range of other energy work methods and techniques, and it is vital to always cleanse and protect before such work, and then cleanse again after. There are all kinds of entities roaming around: good, bad, neutral, weak, and also very powerful. They all have their own agenda, much like people do. Psychic energy is interesting for many of them. It could be seen as a source of energy, food, or simply a light attracting them like a moth. Maybe they wish to protect and help you, but you can't count on that. Some, like your spirit guides, angels, or spirit tribe, are helpful and beneficent. Other entities may be less well intentioned. It might be a little simplistic to say that there is a continual tug of war between light and dark. A human serves as an energetic battery pack of sorts, and a psychic even more so. Empaths vibrate higher and more powerfully than most, and should make sure to protect themselves not just from people, but from entities in the spirit world. Instead of white light, I would use silver light for this. Anything with bad intent does not like seeing its own reflection, so when ill-intentioned spirits approach you, the silver bubble of protection around you not only guards but also repels them and makes it less likely that they will come back for a second look.

Moreover, do not overlook spaces and items and the energy imprint they have. Be aware that:

- Gifts given to you by those who have ill will towards you (or are just toxic people in general) are best not kept at all. Alternatively, you can energetically cleanse them with white light before using.

- Chairs, cutlery, plates, bus seats, office chairs, waiting rooms, and any piece of furniture or equipment that others commonly use needs to be energetically cleansed before you sit on them or touch them. Otherwise you take the chance of absorbing the unwanted energies of those who were there before you. This can be done in seconds, with a quick visualization of cleansing white light around the items.

- Rooms, offices, new houses, and often-frequented spaces all carry an energy. You can clear that, without the extra effort of burning sage all the time. Carry protective crystals or herbs for going outside in general, and clear an area with a visualization of white light and earth energy as needed. If you are a geomantic empath, feel into the energy of the ground of a new place to see if there are bad vibes or pollution. When moving into a new office or home, you can clear the space with clearing room sprays (made up of half vodka, half water, a teaspoon of salt, lavender, and rosemary oil, or whatever plant additives you wish to use. Geranium is also a great cleanser and protector. Use witch hazel instead of vodka if you have pets). You can even go so far as to create and install a permanent, protective crystal grid using black tourmaline, rose or clear quartz, and the like. Or you can supercharge your room spray by making a crystal grid around the spray bottle.

- Avoid touching people or allowing them within your personal bubble unless you choose to have them there. Stay aware of how your energy feels versus theirs, and cleanse after a lot of touching.

These sorts of actions should become second nature to you after a while, but in the beginning, you may need to put a reminder on your phone or calendar.

Grounding your energy is also something you want to make a regular part of your day. You may notice days where you feel scattered—bumping into and knocking over things, catching your clothes on doors and furniture, and having lots of little accidents. This is the universe telling you to slow down and ground yourself. Other signs to get grounded include overthinking, frequent flights of your mind to anywhere except where you are, spacing out, and excessive anxiety.

Some simple grounding techniques include

- Stop moving and concentrate on your body. Stand or sit squarely on the earth. Send your awareness deep down into Mother Earth. Feel the soil, roots, rocks, and grounding energy beneath you and draw on that. You only need to do this for a few minutes at most to feel grounded once again.

- Use your breath to slow yourself down. Breathe slowly to the count of 10. You can also drink a cool glass of water slowly. That automatically slows and calms things.

- Splash your face with cold water.

- Walk on the earth barefoot.

- Carry sprigs of herbs or crystals like black tourmaline, hematite, red jasper, or shungite on you.

- Smell an earthy scent, like fresh soil or the plants in your garden. Turmeric, cinnamon, and garlic are also great scents for grounding you.

If your energy is consistently ungrounded, eat more root vegetables (potatoes, carrots, parsnips, etc.) and mushrooms. Become mindful of moving and speaking just a little bit slower than normal. Focus on the present moment and be as fully aware of it as you can.

Mental and Emotional Mastery

Learning how to control and focus your mind and emotions will naturally boost your psychic abilities.

It helps to know that thoughts lead to feelings. Emotions can sometimes come from physical issues like hunger, illness, chemical or hormonal imbalances, and so on, but don't underestimate the role our thoughts play in how we feel.

Basically, what you allow yourself to think—if you think it often enough—will create either feelings of satisfaction, peace, and joy… or the opposite. This is why it is so important to learn how to curate the quality of your thoughts. Observe and question them as often as needed.

Your emotions power a lot of your psychic strength and feed into your ability to manifest a reality that you want. Attaching positive, strong emotion to your goals and intentions is an extremely powerful way to reinforce them on a subconscious and spiritual level.

Part of mastering your thoughts also requires going inwards and looking at past pain and hurt because this is what often drives our fears, weaknesses, and poor choices. This type of thought mastery is also called shadow work since we are facing our shadow side that is often kept in the dark, avoided, denied, and suppressed.

Practical Exercise: Observe Yourself

For a week or two, carry a pencil and notepad with you wherever you go. When anything goes wrong or you notice that you are feeling bad:

1. Make a note of what just happened.

2. What were you thinking right before you had these feelings?

3. Is there a pattern to these thoughts?

4. What new thoughts would be less destructive to you and more helpful?

5. When you observe your thoughts, use this language, "I notice that I am having a thought that…" See how that helps you step back from it all and deal with it less reactively and judgmentally.

Shadow work sounds mysterious and sexy, but it is actually hard and uncomfortable. Like pricking an abscess so the poison can drain, the wound is lanced and it can heal. If you are brave enough, you can make incredible strides in healing and building overall strength and resilience with shadow work.

It helps to face, accept, and work through past trauma, mistakes, shame, guilt, fears, and pain. Doing this work helps you integrate all the aspects of yourself and work with, not against, yourself. Shadow work stops issues going unresolved or building up inside until they come out undesirable ways. Unresolved shadows express themselves as anger, fear, insecurity, reactive behavior, and poor choices.

First we need to accept that we have a dark side. Only by seeing it and understanding it can we work better with it. We can either then get help, do our own work, or set up systems to help us manage our dark side so that it does not cause us further trouble. There are so many options.

Anything that promotes self-awareness will help you engage with your shadow side better. These activities can include:

- Participating in meditation and reflection
- Attending courses, reading and researching into various issues that can help open up your thinking
- Going to some forms of therapy
- Facing your fears
- Unpacking unhelpful root beliefs and life lessons that you may have internalized as a young child or teen
- Practicing self-love and self-care

Practical Exercise: Shedding Light on the Shadows

Practice noticing when your shadows emerge. This will usually happen during an argument or when you're feeling fearful or insecure. Journal about what you notice:

1. What triggers your fear or anger?
2. What parts of your past do you not like to think about, but you don't believe are healed or resolved?

3. What heavy emotions do you find hard to shake? If you are stuck in an emotion for longer than 5 minutes and can't shake it off, this is a sign that there is an underlying shadow that needs attention

4. What people do you really dislike? Often we have this reaction to others because we see in them a part of ourselves that we do not like.

It may be hard to admit to some of this, but if you are brave and patient with yourself, you will start seeing patterns emerging. Then you can start doing the work to shift any unwanted aspects of yourself. Perfection is not the goal here. Where there is light there will always be some shadow, and perfection is an illusion. Life and growth are a continual shifting journey towards the light, so don't beat yourself up if from time to time shadows creep back. Just do your best. Shadows are part of being human.

Re-parenting Yourself

Think back to your childhood. What experiences stand out for you? How did you feel? What were you most often punished or criticized for? What did you need that you did not get?

Understand that your parents were likely doing their best. Parents make mistakes just like everybody else. So this is not about blaming anyone. This is about taking responsibility for where you are right now and then doing what is necessary to shift towards where you want to go.

One way to know what it is you most need, or needed as a child but did not get, is to look at how you show love and care to others. Gary Chapman, in his 5 Love Languages books, goes into depth about this topic. We show the love that we never had.

Do you show love through (Chapman, 2015):

- Acts of service and doing things for others?
- Kind, heartfelt words of appreciation and encouragement?
- Time spent with someone?
- Physical touch, hugs, caresses, and so on?
- Giving helpful and thoughtful gifts?

Whichever love languages you express are what you need. So how can you start giving yourself love in this way?

Other ways to re-parent that distressed little inner child is to simply ask it what it needs. Picture yourself as a child in your mind's eye, or even find a photograph of yourself from when you were little. Out loud, ask yourself what you need. Then wait patiently because your inner child will answer you. Listen deeply. Keep a box of tissues handy as this exercise can get very emotional.

Think about how what happened in childhood might have affected how you behave, your choices, and how you live your life. Look for unhealthy or unhelpful habits or patterns that you may have carried into adulthood. It is very common for us to learn a survival strategy as a child and then, unconsciously, keep using that same strategy for decades. We may never stop to think that as an adult we have way more choices than we did as a child. Reflecting on this is very useful because you can bring to light so much baggage you have been carrying unnecessarily. In the process, you can choose to put those heavy burdens down.

If you are ready and able, consider forgiveness—for yourself and for your caregivers.

Oprah says, "Forgiveness is giving up the hope that the past could have been any different, it's accepting the past for what it was, and using this moment and this time to help yourself move forward" (GoodReads, n.d). I couldn't say it any better. Forgiveness does not mean agreeing with, excusing, or even forgetting what happened. It just means letting go, taking the lesson, and then putting your energy and attention somewhere else. Living in an unhappy past will only hurt you, not the people who created that situation.

Letting go of hatred, shame, guilt, and the rest is an incredibly freeing, healing, and empowering choice to make. In this way, you can authentically move forward into a future less tainted with the pain of the past.

Chapter 9:
Strengthening Psychic Skills

Out of suffering have emerged the strongest souls; the most massive characters are seared with scars. –Khalil Gibran

Once you have your psychic hygiene and protection in place and feel that these habits have become a strong and regular part of your life, you are at a powerful and safe enough place to take your psychic empath abilities to the next level.

By now, you should be feeling a lot less psychic "interference." You should be able to walk into a crowded room, have a busy "people" day, or even attend a rock concert and not take on anything you don't want to. If that is not yet the case, I recommend going back and spending more time on your protection and energy cleaning practices. Do not go expanding and honing your psychic ability before this. That would be like handing a sharp knife to a toddler and telling them to carve the Sunday roast. You would be asking for trouble.

However, there are two areas you can always work with, even if your ability to protect your energy is still a work in progress: mindfulness and meditation. Both of these techniques are simply life skills that benefit anyone who tries them.

Meditation

You may know all about this. You may even have tried it. But are you doing it regularly?

The point of meditating is not to be all holier-than-thou and super spiritual or to look good. No. The point is that you are training your mind and strengthening mental muscles to be able to be calm and focused at will.

Meditation has many benefits. It is good for mental agility, memory, blood pressure, gut function, and your system as a whole. Why? Because it significantly helps reduce your everyday levels of anxiety, worry, and stress. This, in turn, means less stress chemicals coursing around your brain and body, less wear and tear on your system, better moods, and better life choices. We always do better from a place of safety and calm rather than fear and stress.

You do not need to overthink meditation. You don't need to learn complex poses and hand mudras (finger positions). You do not need special equipment, clothing, or music. You actually need nothing. Just yourself and some uninterrupted time.

There are truly many ways to meditate and none of them are wrong, as long as you apply these principles:

- Don't aim to think of nothing. The harder you try to force this, the less fun it is for you. Also, it is quite impossible- our minds love to` leap around like monkeys at a party. What you need to do is give those monkeys something to do, especially in the early days when you are still training them. Maybe one day your monkeys will all calm down and behave when told, but this cannot happen at the beginning. So here are some calming tools for the monkeys:

- Counting and breathing are my favorites as they are so simple and easy. Counting is reflexive. Most of us can do it without a lot of thought, but it is sufficient to distract the monkey mind. If thoughts intrude, simply let them go and start counting from one again.

- Walking helps your mind focus on where you are putting your feet, so walking meditations can be a lovely way to calm the mind. Just choose a safe path or circuit and mindfully place each step slowly as you walk. Focus on the steps fully. Crunchy gravel or beach sand is nice for this kind of meditation.

- Watch a candle flame.

- Focus on a mandala.

- Use sound, like a healing MHz, mantra, or meditation music.

- Follow a guided meditation. I quite like Oprah and Deepak Chopra's combination meditations for this, but there are plenty available online. You can even record and playback your own words and music, which is quite useful for visualizations and manifestation too.

• Be comfortable. If that means you are lying down, so be it. You don't want your body to distract you from the meditation at first. If you fall asleep, well, that just means you got very relaxed and is not a bad thing

• Decide what to do with your eyes. They do not need to be closed. Open-eye meditation, where you look at some fairly uninteresting point or a mandala or flame, is a good way to train your brain for circumstances in daily life when you want to drop into a state of calm focus and still see where you are and what you are doing. Closed-eyed meditation is helpful when you are trying to visualize something. They are both useful but serve different purposes

There is no perfect or right way to meditate—just what works for you. Start out doing it consistently, at about the same time of day, but don't make it so complicated that you feel put off or overwhelmed. You want to make it easy enough that it feels easy to do no matter what. So start with perhaps only a few minutes a day, and when that starts happening without you having to think about it much, then you can start adding extra time and complexity into the mix.

Mindfulness

Mindfulness also sounds way more complicated than it actually is. Living mindfully is all about being present in the moment. And the reason you want to do this is because now is when life is happening. The past holds memories, which only exist in your head. The past cannot be changed- it can only be learned from.

The future holds hopes, wishes, plans, and desires. But the future is not real yet. It is all in your mind, and perhaps linked to a few things you choose to do right now if you have a plan that you are working towards.

Living in the past can often hold regret or shame, and living in the future only holds worries and anxiety. You can visit the past and future to learn or plan, but never live there because that means you are living in an illusion. While illusions can be pretty or nightmarish, they are not why you are here. They are temporary. They are unreal.

If you wish to live your life fully and richly and to get the most out of each moment, then right here and now is where your attention, awareness, and focus needs to be.

There is a very simple way to be mindful. Just keep asking yourself, "Am I here, now?" That is enough to bring you into the present moment. You can even set a reminder on your phone or device as an alarm or screensaver.

You will not get it 100% right straightaway, but over time, you will find it easier to stay focused in the present.

Psychic Aids

There are many methods of supporting psychic learning journeys. Plants distilled into teas, tinctures, or unguents or even smoked can provide a bridge for the senses and elevate your energetic vibrations, albeit temporarily.

The psychotherapeutic community has discovered that many psychedelic plants and substances have incredible healing properties. They are being used to treat PTSD, anxiety, and major depressive disorder, among other things. The way these chemicals are used, the intention, and the manner in which the experience is integrated back into daily life is what makes the difference between a drug user taking drugs for kicks and someone who gets a real, deep benefit from these substances.

The shamanic community are probably the best ones to access to explore these benefits properly on a psychic level. Their sweat lodges and vision quests can be hugely beneficial.

Herb and plant teachers you can try at home include mugwort, valerian, rosemary, and lavender. Try each, one at a time, and spend a week or so with it. Drink it as a tea or smudge with it. Sit with the plant, if you have a live one, and feel into its energy. See what learning comes from the experience. Especially, look to your dreams. Mugwort in particular is good for this. The Nordic shamans and energy workers love using it. Blue lotus is also interesting, as are angelica and yarrow.

Get Some Help

One thing that helps anyone on the path of psychic and spiritual growth is finding a mentor or teacher. Simply being around a person who is vibrating at a higher energetic level will help elevate you as well.

Each person will have their own specific teachings to share, so don't stick with only one source of learning. In fact, consider searching out local energy work courses, talks, workshops and events and see what each can contribute. Some will be pivotal and others may not, but it is always lovely being in a group of people who are working and living on this level, and you never know where your next flash of insight and knowledge will come from.

I have experienced deep learning from children, animals, and nature. Also, every person I help on my psychic empath journey brings their own wisdom and some sort of learning experience.

Don't be afraid to try new things, meet new people, and forge new bonds. You may even find your tribe in the process.

Chapter 10:

Psychic Awakenings

That is the real spiritual awakening, when something emerges from within you that is deeper than who you thought you were. So, the person is still there, but one could almost say that something more powerful shines through the person.
–Eckhart Tolle

A psychic awakening is quite an alarming thing if you are not prepared for it. It can take you unawares and be quite a painful experience.

Awakenings are triggered by any number of situations, such as major life changes or traumas such as life-threatening illnesses, divorces, car accidents, pandemics, midlife crises, depression or anxiety, or even near-death type of experiences. You can even trigger one on purpose with something like skydiving or, perhaps, a shamanic journey with ayahuasca or similar.

In essence, it is a situation that causes you to rethink yourself and your life. This can lead to mental and spiritual growth. For a psychic, this can also trigger the related psychic growth.

First, you need to understand that this is not a process that happens once and is over. You may experience several over a lifetime although the first one is often the most intense.

Signs That You May Be Awakening

There is a common thread in faith traditions that describes this state as nirvana, enlightenment, or awakening. Consciousness occurs when you stop being the observer and instead ask yourself: who is watching?

The most common signs of awakening include:

- Every once in awhile you suddenly become aware that you are witnessing or observing yourself, as if from a bit of a distance.

- You feel more connected to others and feel a pull towards making some sort of positive change for your fellow humans.

- You find it easier to let go of preconceptions of who you are, which you previously attached a lot of importance to.

- You are more in tune with your intuition.

- Life starts displaying a strange sort of synchronicity and serendipity. Subtle signs start showing up and giving you little hints.

- You are not that scared of the end of your life anymore, but not in a self-sabotaging way.

- You feel an increased need to be who you are, your authentic self. Trying to be anything else is simply exhausting and irritating.

Other signs can include a bit of emotional upheaval. You may have a pre-awakening that involves some anxiety, lightheadedness, strange dreams, and emotions all over the place. Relationships can start shifting and changing. You may feel a little disconnected from mundane life and a bit alone. Your senses may feel heightened, and you may even feel ill with headaches and the like for a little while.

You can even trigger an awakening yourself, mainly through meditation, reflection, breathwork, yoga, and following a diet without meat, alcohol, preservatives and with clean, raw plant matter.

The Process

While yours may take a different form, spiritual gurus have broken down the phases of a spiritual awakening into several steps (Gabriel, 2018):

1. The awakening involves a lot of questioning of the status quo. You may start clearing certain things out of your life, like destructive relationships, old beliefs, and habits.

2. The dark night of the soul is a pretty rough patch. You feel stripped down to the raw. It can be very challenging and sometimes you may feel like you have hit rock bottom. Be assured that this is also the catalyst for some very positive changes even if you can't see it right now.

3. The sponge phase is when you start absorbing new ideas and wisdom and start recreating yourself.

4. The satori phase is when things start falling into place and making more sense.

5. The soul session is when you start rebuilding a firmer life structure based on your new learning.

6. Surrender is releasing the last unhelpful bits of your old self.

7. Service is when you share what you have gained and learned with others, understanding that through service comes real joy and inner peace.

You may even recognize that you are in one of these phases right now.

How to Handle It

If you believe you are in the middle of an awakening, it helps to relax into it as much as possible rather than to resist it. Put whatever support systems in place that you need. Ask for help, rest, and apply self-care on every level.

Look around you for your tribe or for other spiritually awakened people and spend time with them. Read, research, watch clips on various media about spiritual awakening because you never know what will strike the right note for you.

At the end of this phase, you will feel a deeper sense of joy, peace, and maybe even bliss. Life will just seem to come together and get a lot easier. You will have come out the other side with more wisdom, greater strength, and deepened psychic abilities.

Chapter 11:
Working With the Universe

To the mind that is still, the whole universe surrenders. —Lao Tzu

On your psychic journey, it helps to open your mind and senses. Whatever higher power, collective unconscious, or universal energy is out there, it is just waiting for you to tap into it. Knowing how it works will be immeasurably helpful for you.

Universal Laws

These universal laws can be found in the book *The Kybalion: A Study of the Hermetic Philosophy of Ancient Egypt and Greece,* as well as across many faiths and wisdom traditions (Three Initiates, 2020):

1. **The principle of mentalism**: This principle explains the true nature of energy, power, and matter. All is mind, the universe is mental.

2. **The law of divine oneness**: Everything is connected. We can even see this in the world of quantum physics. Whatever you do has an effect on many other things within yourself, possibly with others, and out in the world. Your choices and actions make a difference.

3. **The law of energy or vibration**: Every atom, even subatomic particles, vibrate at various frequencies. Nothing stands still. Objects that vibrate at a similar frequency attract

each other. This is why if you want to manifest a desire, matching your vibration to the thing you want before you have it attracts it to you. Nothing rests. Everything moves. Everything vibrates. This principle explains that the manifestations of matter, energy, mind, and spirit result from varying rates of vibration.

4. **The law of correspondence**: This law states that patterns are everywhere. As above, so below, as within, so without. Smaller patterns often reflect bigger ones. This principle enables one to extrapolate from the known to the unknown.

5. **The law of cause and effect**: This law means that every action has a reaction.

6. **The law of transmutation**: Even the smallest action can have a ripple effect.

7. **The law of compensation**: This law is about reaping what you sow.

8. **The law of attraction**: Life mirrors where you are on an energetic level. If life on the outside seems chaotic or not that great, it is not a punishment, but rather a reflection of what is going on within you. Fortunately, this can be changed. You are capable of making different decisions and attracting a different set of circumstances.

9. **The law of relativity**: Relativity states that in order for us to develop, we have to go through a series of challenges. This is how life unfolds- through mistakes, struggles, and what we overcome.

10. **The law of polarity**: All is duality. Everything has poles; everything has its pairs of opposites; like and unlike are the

same. Opposites are identical but different in degree. Opposites are only two extremes of the same thing, with many varying degrees between.

11. **The law of perpetual motion**: Everything flows out and in. Everything has its tides; all things rise and fall. The pendulum swing manifests in everything, rhythm compensates. This principle of neutralization applies in the affairs of the Universe, suns, worlds; in life, mind, energy, matter. There is always an action and a reaction, an advance and a retreat.

12. **The principle of gender**: Gender is in everything—everything has its masculine and feminine principles. Gender manifests on all planetary levels. Everything and everyone contains the same two principles within them—him or her.

These simple principles unlock the mysteries of matter-energy, spirit-mind, and consciousness. Through them, a profound transformation of conscious life can be achieved. This book is an argument for undertaking such a journey, demonstrating that transformation on the mental and energetic planes will have immediate consequences in the material realm. Each principle affects the others in a reciprocal manner, ensuring cohesion and unity of the multifaceted universe.

Subconscious and Superconscious

Higher energies do not speak using the common tongue or any language we know. Possibly the closest link may be found in ancient Sanskrit, but as frustrating as it may seem, it helps to understand that while the universe may be trying to communicate with you, it cannot do this using words directly.

This is why even the ancient Greek oracles spoke in symbols and images because this is how the universe speaks. We can tune in to the universe in dreams, visions, patterns, and symbols. Psychic readers tune in to it via the tarot, rune stones, or other reading tools. The tools are not what do the trick; they simply provide a way for us to receive universal messages that we may otherwise be unlikely to pick up on.

Probably the easiest way to receive messages is via your dreams. You can look up dream symbology, but the best way to interpret your dreams is to ask yourself what each symbol means to you. Some symbols have universal meaning, but others are specific to certain cultures and backgrounds, which is why you really cannot apply a universal dictionary to them.

Practical Exercise: Reading Your Dreams

Keep a notepad and pencil next to your bed. On waking do not hesitate to write down what you remember because you will forget otherwise. If you struggle to remember dreams, drink a glass of water before bed. This tends to wake you more often (to go pee) and makes it more likely you will wake during or right after REM (rapid eye movement) sleep, which is when you tend to dream.

1. What main images were in your dreams?
2. What colors did you notice?
3. Who was there?
4. What places did you notice?
5. What feelings did you have about any of the dream?

The most important thing to consider is what each of these answers specifically means to you.

Empaths dream a little differently from others. We tend to have very vivid dreams that we recall more easily than normal. We may have more nightmares too. Some empaths have lucid dreams where we are conscious that we are, in fact, dreaming. Once you can relax into lucid dreaming, this is a very useful skill because you can approach the dream with an air of curiosity rather than shock or fear.

Connecting to Your Spirit Guides

Anything you do that raises your vibrations will help with this connection. Meditating, showing gratitude, eating a diet that causes no harm to other living beings, avoiding alcohol and toxic chemicals, being in nature, and maintaining psychic hygiene will all help.

You can visualize a meeting and see what comes up, or you can do a shamanic spirit journey to connect. You can ask for a sign, or request a message, answer, or connection in the dream world. You can even speak your wishes, questions, or hopes out loud, and then wait and see what comes up. Your guides are just waiting for a chance to connect, so if you make yourself available, they certainly will be there for you.

Chapter 12:
Out in the World

Let us be grateful to people who make us happy, they are the charming gardeners who make our souls blossom. –Marcel Proust

Most empaths will agree that getting out and about and spending time with people is not at the top of their list. It's not that we do not like others. We may, in fact, be quite extroverted in many ways, although this normally comes in the form of an extroverted introvert who enjoys occasional socializing but still needs to retreat at times to re-energize and recharge. This type of approach becomes more possible once we have our psychic hygiene and protection routines firmly in place.

Telling Others

Before you tell anyone who or what you are, get clear on why you need to tell them anything at all. If it's just to make you feel good about yourself, it's probably best to find another way to do that. There are some people who just delight in crashing into conversations and dropping the gem that they are, indeed, an empath. This is seldom the best way to open up a dialogue. There are better ways to talk about what it means to be an empath.

Consider what sort of person you are speaking with. Do they seem open-minded, empathetic, kind, respectful, or interested (for the right reasons)? Not everyone can be trusted or needs to know that much about you. I prefer to err on the side of caution, and I actually seldom use the word "empath" when describing myself. Those that I assist with healing and energy work naturally know what my nature is anyway.

There is nothing wrong with using the label when advertising your skills if you want to create a commercial venture out of who you are and your abilities. I know many animal whisperers, energy workers, readers, and teachers who never hesitate to say exactly what they are. Psychic empaths using their abilities in this way are more than encouraged to ask for energy exchanges in the form of cash for their time and energy. We all need to eat, after all.

When you tell others about your nature, consider why you are telling them and, thus, how much information they need. For example, if you are doing healing work, you can choose to tell your clients how you are able to feel into their energy, or not. I know a high profile therapist who mostly keeps things fairly mainstream, but for those clients who indicate they are open to understanding more and working on an energetic level, she adds this dimension into their therapy plan. For the others, she still uses her skills to get a better reading of where they are at, but she simply doesn't tell them because she knows many people would find that information distracting and confusing. They may also immediately stigmatize her and take their business elsewhere.

Smoothing Over Close Relationships

When you are around certain people more than others, they may have questions or want to understand you better. Again you can choose how much you tell them.

At work, for example, I would limit these types of conversations to people who are able to process this kind of information. Otherwise, you might find your life and career limited by unhelpful preconceptions and stereotypes. It is better that they simply think that you are moody than they think you are moody and irrational, for example. If you learn to manage and protect your energies, then no one really needs to know anything. All they may notice, in this case, is that you are very perceptive and have an uncanny knack for knowing things, which will gain you a lot of respect. Often those who are open to knowing more will have already guessed what sort of person you are all by themselves anyway.

A classic example of this that I see in my own life is when I move into a new neighborhood. Without me saying a word, people start gravitating towards me. They notice my herbal cupboard (if I have invited them in) and also my healthy family and my way with animals. They listen to my responses to their questions and often this quickly escalates into them asking for my advice on any range of topics. Before long, I will have some of them tentatively approaching me and cautiously asking if I can help them with problems that fall outside the realm of "normal." I may find myself mixing healing herbal teas and doing energy work without ever having to say a single thing about who or what I am. It's kind of amusing.

In romantic relationships, my advice is to be completely honest about all things including this. Maybe not on your very first date, but a couple dates in, you should be able to open up more. If the person is unable to comprehend what a psychic empath is or blocks themselves to this level of knowledge, then they really aren't the kind of person you should be in a relationship with in the first place. Trust, openness, and the ability to see and be seen are the building blocks for a sound life partnership. Even better, someone who can walk this spiritual path with you would be an ideal partner.

Setting Boundaries

Although we have already spoken about boundaries in their basic sense earlier in the book, psychic boundaries are a little different and need some extra attention.

Before going out to work or into any social situation, it's best to pull in your auric field and close down your chakras. Don't forget to cleanse and reopen yourself up when you are back in a safe space. Put your protections in place like clockwork before you step outside your front door. This is your first and most important boundary.

Practice saying no because you are going to need it. Empaths give off such a beautiful, comforting energy that people are naturally drawn to us. They want to be close to us, touch us, hug us, and, well, that's a problem for us more than for them, of course. I, for one, can get worried about total strangers having toxic or chaotic energy when they are near me. I maintain a personal bubble of about a meter at the very least. Also, I am not above raising my hand, palm out, sometimes in a vague way, and placing it subtly between me and an oncoming space invader. This is quite a powerful gesture and stops most people in their tracks.

Of course, there are times, like at a rock concert, in a queue, or on a subway train or bus, that people get way closer than you would like. But you have your protections in place, and you can do a thorough clearing of yourself as soon as you are away from the crush. You can also simply take up more space. Stand with your feet wide apart and your elbows out, for starters. Don't be afraid to firmly move people away from you if needed or even to say out loud, "Excuse me, please give me some space."

Wearing headphones (even if nothing is playing) is one way to get some peace and quiet. Or carrying and reading a book can help- although I don't often take a book to a concert.

Women especially are taught to be polite, but there is no way I am going to stand docilely while someone rubs himself against my back on a metro or subway train. I will speak up and loudly too- even if it's just a firm "excuse me!" If you don't protect your boundaries, it is unlikely that anyone else will.

There is also the skill of sheer presence of will. As you develop your psychic abilities and willpower, you may notice that you find it easier to repel unwanted space invaders with the sheer power of your presence and intent. This is a handy skill to work on. You don't need to say anything—just focus your energy on a general "back off" or "go away" and see what happens.

Chapter 13:

Using Your Gifts

Anybody who succeeds is helping people. The secret to success is to find a need and fill it; find a hurt and heal it; find a problem and solve it. –Robert H. Schuller

Just because you have these special abilities does not mean you have to do anything with them. However, it would be a bit of a waste if you chose to shut yourself down and shut your abilities out.

Many wisdom traditions agree that the highest act of love is service. How you choose to give that service is up to you. It could be random acts of kindness or simply letting others know that you see and understand them to some degree. But you are capable of so much more.

When you start developing your abilities, once you know where your psychic empath strengths lie, this will give you some indication of what else you can do with your gifts.

Good Help vs. Bad Help

Being of service means that you are helping others in some way. As a psychic empath, you are lucky enough to have certain skills most other people do not. But, as we know, with great power comes great responsibility. Before you go barging in to save the day, consider the following:

- Does the person (or plant/animal) you wish to help actually want your help, or any help? You cannot change, improve, shift, or heal where it is unwanted. This is, in fact, crossing another's boundaries in an unhealthy way if you force help on them.

- Have they asked you for help? If it is a non-verbal being, you can feel a clear yes or no before you begin helping randomly.

- What is your intention with the help you are giving? Is it to actually make a positive difference in the world, or is it to make you look good, make your life easier, or assuage some guilt you have?

- Is your help going to empower them to move forward after you have aided them, on their own and without you? Good help uplifts, inspires, heals, and empowers others. This is the difference between teaching a person to fish and giving them a fish. If your help makes another dependent on you and they are not your child or your pet, it is probably not a healthy arrangement.

- Is your help going to help them achieve their own sense of purpose and direction rather than one you think they should be following?

If your help undermines a person's strength, self-determination, independence, and confidence, then it is not a good sort of help, and it is best to stop or never even start in the first place.

It may be hard for empaths because our natural tendency is to save the world and everything in it, but we have to resist the urge and first check ourselves at the door. Otherwise we stand to create more harm than good.

The wrong kind of help given will, more often than not, backfire on you in some way. You will fall out with the people you are trying to help; they may grow to dislike or even hate you, or you may end up with a permanent taker who just loves that they have found someone to leech off of.

Empath Careers

You will find empaths in all walks of life, doing any number of things- although quite often the act of service will be involved somehow.

Geopaths and earth empaths are often found in environmental conservation, preservation, or in professions such as dowsing, surveying, or even construction. They may find themselves working with clay, foraging for wild edibles, caring for a forest or river land, farming, or pretty much anything to do with the land. That is what their skills set them up for, really. And the land always responds so well to them too.

Plant empaths will fall into similar professions and may find themselves running a plant nursery or doing botany, herbology, forestry, or farming.

Animal empaths make great vets, animal whisperers, and farmers as well.

Precogs can be found in corporate boardrooms working on organizational strategy, or they may prefer a quieter life running a small psychic reading/energy work business.

Telepaths and intuitives can be found literally anywhere and everywhere. This skill works for you no matter what you do. The world is your oyster.

Dream and emotive empaths are often found in mental therapy fields or as some sort of healer, shaman, or energy worker offering these services to others.

Always consider what your abilities are enabling you to do. Where do your strengths lie and how can you use them for your own higher good, the good of mankind, and the world at large? Because you are a psychic empath, it is quite easy for these answers to come to you. Check in with your energy and feelings around possible career paths, and your gut will tell if your spirit guides don't.

Chapter 14:
Parenting an Empath Child

There's nothing more satisfying than seeing a happy and smiling child. I always help in any way I can... A child's smile is worth more than all the money in the world. –Lionel Messi

Psychic empath abilities can often run in families. But an untrained, unsupported empath can also easily be pushed over into major depression, anxiety, or other personality disorders if they experience sufficient trauma early on. Unfortunately, it is not hard for this to happen when a small soul is fragile, unprotected, and vulnerable.

Most parents do not want any harm of any kind for their children. But some parents have their own dysfunctions and pain to sort through, so they inadvertently pass this on to their children, along with psychic abilities. It is up to each individual whether they choose to heal and grow, to break the cycle of pain and suffering, or to perpetuate it.

We all operate from the level that we are at. We do what we can with the knowledge and resources that we have at the time. Sometimes these are more limited, and we make mistakes. If you have chosen to have children, hopefully you are intent on making as few mistakes as possible. That being said, you will still make some mistakes—that is a given. Your child will still experience some form of challenge and hardship because that is life. You just hope that you don't contribute too much to that.

No matter what, there will be a time when a very young empath is picking up on other people's feelings (and more) but does not yet realize this fact. They absorb the emotional energy all around them and experience a strange emotional roller coaster. They think all these emotions are theirs alone, and it can be a very confusing and exhausting time. Sometimes they may be diagnosed with major depression, anxiety, bipolar, or borderline personality disorder, among other things.

If you are reading this book, the odds are that you are the kind of parent that is more self-aware and conscious, that you are working on yourself, and that you are aware of how your actions impact your children and want to make sure their experience with you is as constructive, safe, and positive as possible.

Signs Your Child Is an Empath

Look out for the early signs. If you know you are a psychic empath, the odds are that your children may be too. But it is not always the case. Genetics can randomly combine and throw out a young person with no psychic empath abilities, and that is okay too.

The main reason you want to watch out for the signs is so that you can help your child avoid the same pain and suffering you may have gone through before you realized what you were and how to manage it. By helping them, you are not limiting their learning opportunities, just limiting the damage that they will later have to work through.

Contrary to popular opinion, learning does not only come through adversity (although this is how it often happens). It can also occur from a base of love.

Common signs to watch out for include

- Your child displays emotional sensitivity and difficulty processing emotions. Children need to be taught emotional intelligence no matter what, but it may be more pronounced with a child empath.

- Your child needs a lot of alone time and feels happier in nature than at a party.

- Your child may be touch adverse. They may dislike being around certain people, or even dislike something as simple as rough textures.

- They may have a special affinity for plants or animals.

- They may like or dislike certain places and not be able to explain why.

- They may scream and cry when specific people approach them, when there is no overt or obvious reason for this. This is commonly seen with empath babies.

The same signs that apply to you will ultimately apply to them. But when they are still very young, they may have trouble verbalizing or explaining what is going on inside them, so the above indicators are useful to know in any case.

Some empathic children may be diagnosed with sensory processing disorder, ADHD, or autism. Behind these labels may lie a deeper story that mainstream doctors will not be tuning in to- but you can.

How to Teach Them and Protect Them

As the parent, you are also the buffer, the teacher, and the care giver. You are your child's biggest and best supporter. And in their early years, you are the one who helps them learn how to process emotions and helps set boundaries for them until they are old enough to do these things for themselves.

Consider adding the following to your parenting strategy:

- Put protections in place for your child and teach them how as they grow in understanding and ability.

- Help your child to identify their energy as separate from others and to know how their own energy feels.

- Put strong boundaries in place for them, and when they are old enough, show them how to know what their own boundaries are and how to set them up. Even if these boundaries are set with you too, a good parent understands that their child is a unique individual who has the right to decide their own path, likes, dislikes, goals, and so forth. You are there to protect them, and that includes protecting their freedom as long as they aren't harming themselves or others

- Limit their social calendars and extracurricular activities. Keep their young life as simple as possible in the early years.

- Take them outdoors and into nature as much as possible since this provides an organic, natural way for them to decompress and equalize.

- Manage the noise. If you know you are going into a busy, social situation, put systems in place to help them. Don't let everyone play pass-the-baby with them. Limit who has access to them, and never force any form of contact with family, friends, or strangers. If possible, don't take them into crowds or into busy stores, but leave them at home with a trusted caregiver, or babysitter.

- Watch for signs of overwhelm and help remove them from the triggering events or people. Take them off for a walk, go jump in puddles, or sit quietly in a room with a book if needed.

- Believe them. Listen to them. Encourage them to tell you how they are feeling from day to day, and make discussions about emotions and thoughts a daily family bonding practice.

- Teach them how to deal with unhelpful labels and stigma. Give them some snappy comebacks, social techniques, and tools that help ease their journey through life.

My son exhibited signs of being a psychic empath very early on. I was lucky in that I was educated enough and ready to help him from day one. I have come to understand my little empath through education, practice, and lots of cuddles. Though he sometimes struggles with the weight of the world, he is one of the most fiercely loving people I have ever known. You are likely exhausted if you have a child who is an empath, but you are also so, so lucky.

Chapter 15:
Tips and Tricks For When Everything Feels Hard

Life is a series of punches. It presents a lot of challenges. It presents a lot of hardship, but the people that are able to take those punches and are able to move forward are the ones that really do have a lot of success and have a lot of joy in their life and have a lot of stories to tell, too. –Josh Turner

If you are lucky enough to get a bunch of empaths together in a room, before long the same song will be sung. Being an empath is challenging, and we all have some fairly common issues we are faced with and need to overcome. Learning how other empaths do it can be useful. Other empaths can give us different perspectives and frames of reference. You don't know what you don't know. Maybe sharing other people's experiences and how they manage their lives can give you some insight you never had before. Here are some bonus tips and tricks I've gotten from other empaths:

- Other people's emotions can turn your day on its head, even if you are the most well-trained empath, and especially if you are having a busy or chaotic day yourself. That is when your protections may be down or you simply forgot to do what you know you need to do. Just remind yourself to check in, ground, clear, and protect at the soonest chance you get.

- You get tired really quickly. Holding boundaries in place and dealing with other people's emotions, as well as a range of extra input from your environment, are exhausting. Rest often, and watch your blood sugar levels. You can always carry healthy snacks, as well as some candy, for serious energy dips.

- Sometimes you will feel burdened by all the compassion you feel. There are so many people needing healing and help, and you simply can't help them all. Step back and choose where to put your energies. Your first choice should always be yourself and your loved ones.

- People are always inviting you to social events. In fact, your calendar books weeks in advance quite often. Generally you feel an incredible drag just getting out of the front door. You need to have at least a few healthy relationships. Social connections are important for us on a human level. But you can also curate your invites and say no whenever you want to.

- Not everyone will understand your need to be alone from time to time. Some people take it personally and get upset. Remind yourself that this reaction is all about their own insecurities, and don't let them guilt you into doing things you don't have the energy for. Good friends will make an effort to understand, and the rest don't matter.

- You need time in between things, events, tasks, and so on. Allow a bit of extra time for these transitions, and don't judge yourself when you feel a little hollow, rushed, or overwhelmed. This is a good time to ground yourself and apply some self-care.

- Sometimes you just feel anxious or really low for no real reason. This can be a result of emotional overwhelm or fatigue or due to the fact you have taken on someone else's energy by accident. Also, being that much more aware of all the pain and suffering in the world around you can be quite a downer at times. See this as an indication that you need some TLC. Find another empath to unload to and practice your self-care that we outlined earlier for you. Expressing what is on your mind, whether through verbalizing it, through art, music, or even journaling it, will all help you with this. Once you have expressed and released these heavy emotions, then turn your focus towards something nicer.

- Some people try to take advantage of your kindness or try to feed off your energy. They use your compassion to manipulate you. Just watch out for this behavior. You know it is a possibility, just like scammers exist in day-to-day life, so they abound on an energetic and psychic level too. Go back to your boundaries, and get clear on who you choose to help, who you don't, and why.

- Narcissists, energy vampires, and troubled souls are drawn to you like moths to a flame. You do not have to allow them into your life. Once you are familiar with the signs, you will find it easier to ward them off from the get-go.

- You get pulled into other people's problems quickly and sometimes before you can take a breath to say no. When you realize this is what has happened, it's a good time to vocalize that "no." It is never too late to withdraw.

- You care a lot about almost everything, and even the smallest thing can set you off. Allow yourself time and space to process these feelings, and don't invalidate or dismiss them, or else they linger even longer.

- It's probably unhealthy for you to watch the news or a horror movie. They are just too disturbing. I refuse to watch any horror movies or even read scary books. I also limit my media exposure and news intake to twice a week at mid-day, and I only skim the headlines unless there is something I really do need to pay more attention to.

Being an empath comes with so many pluses. As you progress with your studies, work on your hygiene and protections and get stronger at the process of just being an empath, you will find any drawbacks get a lot more manageable.

I know so many happy, stable, successful empaths who have put their abilities to good use for themselves and others and I know it is possible to find peace and enjoy a good quality of life. You just need to do a little work first.

Conclusion

Learning to stand in somebody else's shoes, to see through their eyes, that's how peace begins. And it's up to you to make that happen. Empathy is a quality of character that can change the world. –Barack Obama

Throughout my years as a practicing empath, psychic, animal whisperer, and reiki practitioner, the thought that there are so many empaths out there who have yet to realize who and what they are has deeply saddened me. These are people who may be suffering unnecessarily due to stigma, stereotypes, and as a result of the common problems and learning curves many empaths go through.

I believe we are an incredible resource for this planet. We are the healers. We are the glue that helps society function better, the peacemakers, the helpers. We deserve a lot more honor and support than we currently get, but I believe that that is also coming. Maybe not in our lifetimes, but there is a definite move towards spiritual and energetic consciousness that can be seen globally. And that gives me hope.

In the meantime, we need to help ourselves and help each other. We need to use our abilities to notice and reach out to other empaths and to give them a helping hand. Also, we need to be mindful of our children, because they too may be continuing the tradition, having genetically inherited our very same abilities.

Our role on this earth is to calm, soothe, and heal suffering. We are perfectly set up with the skills we need to do so if we can only heal ourselves first.

It may take us some time to realize what is going on. Social stigma, misconceptions, and an abundance of people walking about with unresolved pain adds to the problem. Toxic positivity and the aversion people have these days towards emotions cuts them off from reading the vital signs and signals they need to improve their lives and heal their own pain. We tend to avoid, suppress, deny, and pretend that we have no emotions, and in the process, we cut ourselves off from an incredibly useful life tool and set of skills. This kind of behavior simply perpetuates suffering as very little gets faced and processed properly, and so it just carries on, bursting out of us at unexpected moments in anger, fear, and other bad choices that create further pain in ourselves and those around us.

Many psychic empaths come to a slow awareness of what they are and how to manage it. And by then, they may have fallen prey to all sorts of energy vampires, narcissists, and other damaged individuals. These individuals cling on to us hoping we can save them, but we cannot. Not until we learn how to save ourselves first.

Learning how to master our minds, our emotions, and our energies is key to stepping into our full power. This is the only way we can let go of our emotional pain and challenges, which may have been following us around until now.

Once you empower yourself, heal yourself, and grow into your full abilities, you open up a huge range of possibilities for yourself. You then get to decide how to use the incredible skills and talents that you have. Our mere presence, being souls who vibrate at a higher level energetically, can influence the energy of our family, workplace, and entire neighborhood. We can uplift and energize just by being there.

You have the option to create such positive shifts in the people and the world around you. Indeed, even small acts of goodness and healing will have a ripple effect. The Universal Laws tell us this is true, and I have seen this in action with my own eyes so many times.

So my hope is that with this book I have given you something to start working on and with. I hope you find useful, practical tools that will help you learn to distinguish yourself and your energy from the energetic noise and chaos around you. I've hopefully given you methods that resonated with you so that you can let go of victimhood, self-hatred, and self-sabotage, and embrace a different kind of future—one that holds joy, peace, and lots of love of all kinds.

This is my wish for you and for every psychic empath out there. We, the healers, also need healing. We need the strength and resilience to do the tasks we have been set on this earth to do.

If my book has helped you, please share it with others who you may know that also need this boost. By leaving a review, you help spread the word to those who may desperately need it too.

We, the psychic empaths of the world, will be watching your growth with love and hope. Reach out to us for a helping hand because you are not alone.

Good luck and safe travels on your journey, you amazing soul you!

Thank You

Thanks so much for purchasing this book and reading to the end. I really appreciate your support and sincerely hope this book has been helpful to you.

There are many books out there on this topic but you chose this one and I am very grateful.

So, from the bottom of my heart, THANK YOU.

Before you go, there's one small favor I wanted to ask you. **If you could consider leaving a review on the platform, it would really help me out. Leaving a review is one of the best and simplest ways to support books from independent authors like me.**

Your feedback is really important to me. It will help me to continue writing books like these to support people like yourself. It would mean a great deal to me to hear from you. I read each and every review posted.

References

Chapman, G. & Green, J. (2017). *The 5 love languages: The secret to love that lasts.* Northfield Publishing.

Clairvoyance quotes (27 quotes). (n.d.). GoodReads. https://www.goodreads.com/quotes/tag/clairvoyance

Cohen, D., Palti, Y., Cuffin, B. N., & Schmid, S. J. (1980). Magnetic fields produced by steady currents in the body. *Proceedings of the National Academy of Sciences,* 77(3), 1447–1451. https://doi.org/10.1073/pnas.77.3.1447

Dandapani. (2019, February 27). *Developing willpower.* https://dandapani.org/blog/developing-willpower/

Empath Quotes (108 quotes). (n.d.). GoodReads. https://www.goodreads.com/quotes/tag/empath

Ewens, H. (2018, November 8). *Super empaths are real, says study.* Vice. https://www.vice.com/en/article/xwj84k/super-empaths-are-real-says-study

Field, Tiffany, et al. (2007, September). Depressed mothers' newborns show less discrimination of other newborns' cry sounds. *Infant Behavior and Development*, 30(3), 431–435. www.doi.org/10.1016/j.infbeh.2006.12.011

Gabriel, R. (2018, December 6). *The 7 stages of spiritual development.* Chopra. www.chopra.com/articles/the-7-stages-of-spiritual-development.

Josh Turner quotes. (n.d.). BrainyQuote.
https://www.brainyquote.com/quotes/josh_turner_515801

Khalil Gibran quotes. (n.d.). BrainyQuote.
https://www.brainyquote.com/quotes/khalil_gibran_386848?src=t_strength

Lao Tzu quotes. (n.d.). BrainyQuote.
https://www.brainyquote.com/quotes/lao_tzu_133381

MacGillivray, L. (2009). I feel your pain: Mirror neurons and empathy. *McMaster University Medical Journal*, 6(1), 16-20. https://mdprogram.mcmaster.ca/docs/default-source/MUMJ-Library/v6_16-20.pdf

Mads Mikkelsen quotes. (n.d.). BrainyQuote.
https://www.brainyquote.com/quotes/mads_mikkelsen_707030?src=t_psychic

Meister Eckhart quotes. (n.d.). BrainyQuote.
https://www.brainyquote.com/quotes/meister_eckhart_149160?src=t_know_yourself

Milstead, K. (2018, July 30). *New research may support the existence of empaths*. Psych Central. https://psychcentral.com/blog/new-research-may-support-the-existence-of-empaths#1

Morris, C. (2017, July 14). *Emotional contagion: Everything you need to know*. Www.issup.net. https://www.issup.net/knowledge-share/resources/2019-11/emotional-contagion-everything-you-need-know

National Childbirth Trust. (2019, June 25). *Empathy for beginners: when do babies tune in to others' thoughts and feelings?* https://www.nct.org.uk/baby-toddler/toddler-tantrums-and-tricky-behaviour/empathy-for-beginners-when-do-babies-tune-others-thoughts-and-feelings

Netz, Y. (2017). Is the comparison between exercise and pharmacologic treatment of depression in the clinical practice guideline of the American College of Physicians evidence-based? *Frontiers in Pharmacology*, 8(257). https://doi.org/10.3389/fphar.2017.00257

Nguyen, J. (2020, May 19). Why everyone's talking about love languages these days & how to find yours. Mindbodygreen. https://www.mindbodygreen.com/articles/the-5-love-languages-explained

Orloff, J. (2018, March 21). *5 scientific explanations of empathy and empaths.* Chopra. https://chopra.com/articles/5-scientific-explanations-of-empathy-and-empaths

Pangilinan, J. (2021, March 24). *45 empath quotes to show your sensitive personality.* Happier Human. https://www.happierhuman.com/empath-quotes/

A quote by Oprah Winfrey. (n.d.). GoodReads. https://www.goodreads.com/quotes/376558-forgiveness-is-giving-up-the-hope-that-the-past-could

A quote by Robert A. Heinlein. (n.d.). GoodReads. https://www.goodreads.com/quotes/125758-everything-is-theoretically-impossible-until-it-is-done-one-could

Ramachandran, V. (n.d.). *The neurons that shaped civilization.* Www.ted.com. https://www.ted.com/talks/vilayanur_ramachandran_the_neurons_that_shaped_civilization?language=en

Riess, H. (2017). The science of empathy. *Journal of Patient Experience,* 4(2), 74–77. https://doi.org/10.1177/2374373517699267

Robert H. Schuller quotes. (n.d.). BrainyQuote. https://www.brainyquote.com/quotes/robert_h_schuller_700700

Scott, E. (n.d.). *Highly sensitive person traits that create more stress.* Verywell Mind. https://www.verywellmind.com/highly-sensitive-persons-traits-that-create-more-stress-4126393

Simpson, E. A., Murray, L., Paukner, A., & Ferrari, P. F. (2014). The mirror neuron system as revealed through neonatal imitation: presence from birth, predictive power and evidence of plasticity. *Philosophical Transactions of the Royal Society B: Biological Sciences,* 369(1644), 20130289. https://doi.org/10.1098/rstb.2013.0289

Three Initiates. (2012). *Kybalion.* Bottom Of The Hill Publis.

Printed in Great Britain
by Amazon